CANCELLED
JUL 23 '7
AF683750
THIS ITEM IS NO LONGER
PROPERTY OF THE
JOHN CRERAR LIBRARY - 1984
8.0852
X902

TISSUE CULTURES

MONOGRAPHS ON ATHEROSCLEROSIS

Vol. 1

Editors:
Henry S. Simms, Rockleigh, New Jersey, USA
John Esben Kirk, St. Louis, Missouri, USA
Otakar J. Pollak, Dover, Delaware, USA

BASEL (Switzerland) S. KARGER NEW YORK

TISSUE CULTURES

O. J. Pollak, M. D., Ph. D.
The Dover Medical Research Center, Inc., Dover, Delaware, USA

Foreword by H. S. Simms

With 28 figures comprising 49 black and white
and 32 color illustrations, 9 tables

1969

BASEL (Switzerland) S. KARGER NEW YORK

Originally published by S. Karger AG, Basel, Switzerland
Distributed exclusively in North America by
THE WILLIAMS & WILKINS COMPANY, BALTIMORE

S. Karger, Arnold-Böcklin-Strasse 25, CH-4000 Basel 11 (Switzerland)

All rights, including that of translation into other languages, reserved.
Photomechanic reproduction (photocopy, microcopy) of this book or parts thereof without special permission of the publishers is prohibited.

©

Copyright 1969 by S. Karger AG, Basel
Printed in Switzerland by Buchdruckerei Gasser AG, Basel
Blocks by Steiner & Co., Basel

CONTENTS

ACKNOWLEDGEMENTS

The author's investigations in the field of Tissue Cultures in Atherosclerosis were made possible by

the financial support of The Delaware Heart Association, Inc., Wilmington, Delaware; The Dover Medical Research Center, Inc., Dover, Delaware; The Lilly Research Laboratories, Eli Lilly and Co., Indianapolis, Indiana; The National Heart Institute, National Institutes of Health, United States Public Health Service, Bethesda, Maryland; The Tobacco Industry Research Committee, New York, New York;

the close collaboration of Minoru Adachi, M.D., Tamako Adachi, M.D., Donald A. Burns, Ph.D., Araceli F. Engel, Ph.D., Tatsuo Kasai, M.D., Reizo Koide, M.D., Tatsuo Kokubu, M.D., Shigeo Nagasawa, M.D., and Akira Wada, M.D.;

the assistance of Joyce N. Budna, B.S., Joan M. Chamberlin, B.S., Bonnie Johanssen, B.S., Patricia Morrow, B.S., Martha Steward, B.S., and Evangelina Z. Vitug, B.S.

The publication of this monograph was made possible with the financial aid from the Dover Medical Research Center, Inc., which allowed reproduction of color illustrations,

with the patient and efficient cooperation of Perry P. Pollak, wife and histologist, Tim Pollak, son and editorial advisor, and Marie Reynolds, secretary and typist.

To the granting agencies, professional collaborators and assistants, co-workers who helped with the manuscript, co-editors of Atherosclerosis Monographs, and to the publisher of the Monograph Series, the author offers his sincerest thanks.

FOREWORD

When living cells were first maintained *in vitro* by Ross Harrison in 1907, the full possibilities of tissue cultures were not anticipated. It was Carrel and Burrows who in 1910 developed the tissue culture as a useful research tool. Others—including Ebeling, Fisher, and Baker—contributed pioneering efforts.

At its birth, the discipline was plagued with technical problems—the necessity for sterility, the selection of optimal biologic nutrients, the use and abuse of growth-promoting embryonic extracts, the maintenance of a proper gas phase. Originally, tissue culture workers concentrated on cell division and migration—on cell growth. Therefore, early studies were made largely on embryonic and neoplastic tissues. But the results from such substrates could not be extrapolated to normal adult tissues.

In time, the technical difficulties were overcome. Synthetic nutrients became available. Pure cell lines could be maintained *in vitro* for long periods. The interest of scientists shifted from cell growth to cell morphology and metabolism. Cells from intact and diseased tissues are now being compared. The transformation of normal cells into altered cells, and the reverse process, have become prime research targets.

Adult cells in an *in vitro* environment never correspond exactly with *in vivo* cells. Nevertheless, in spite of the contrived environment of the tissue culture, such research has led to important and valid observations. Our knowledge of neoplastic growth has increased considerably through tissue culture work. More recently, tissue culture methods have been used in the investigation of atherosclerosis.

The editors of 'Monographs on Atherosclerosis', while striving to be informative and accurate, must bear in mind the influence which they have on scientific terminology. In this volume, the author has attempted to correct the often vague nomenclature of atherosclerosis literature. He uses the word 'lipoid'—instead of the improperly derived 'lipid'—to refer to fat and fat-like substances. He uses the correct designation 'fibrocyte'—frequently though not consistently—since the commonly applied term 'fibroblast' implies a primitive cell. He prefers the term 'myocyte' to the often used 'smooth muscle cell', for there are no striated cells in the vessel wall. He avoids the term 'foam cell'—except in direct quotation from a reference—since it applies to an artifact produced during the preparation of tissues for microscopic study. Instead, the author refers to such cells as 'fat-laden macrophages', where the origin is known, or to 'fat-laden cells', where the origin is uncertain.

The author of this text, Dr. O. J. POLLAK, is an experienced researcher in atherosclerosis. In the last decade, he and his associates have made meritorious contributions to the development and utilization of tissue cultures in atherosclerosis. By combining *in vitro* and *in vivo* experiments, Dr. POLLAK has elucidated the basic etiologic factors of atherogenesis. His broad knowledge of the field qualifies him as a critical reviewer of the literature on tissue cultures in atherosclerosis. I am confident that the reader will consider his endeavors worthwhile.

June 1969 HENRY S. SIMMS

LIST OF ABBREVIATIONS

ADP, AMP, ATP – adenosine di-, mono- tri-phosphate
CPIB – ethyl-α-p-chlorophenoxyisobutyrate
CS, CSC – cigarette smoke, cigarette smoke condensate
CS-A, CS-B, CS-C – chondroitinsulfate A, B, C
DN, FT – denicotinized, filter-tipped
DNA, RNA – desoxyribonucleic acid, ribonucleic acid
DPH – diphenylhydramine HCl
EE – embryo extract
F^2, F^3, .. – second, third, .. generation
GV – growth values
MPS – mucopolysaccharides
NEFA – nonesterified fatty acids
PABA – paraaminobenzoic acid
SDH – succinic dehydrogenase
UF – ultrafiltrate

Cell Strains

BM III – mouse lymphoblasts
HeLa – cervical cancer cells
L-929 – mouse fibroblasts
L-5179Y – mouse leukemia lymphoblasts

Nutrients

199 – Morgan's et al.
BME – basal medium, Eagle's
HMA-4 – Spinner's
MB 752/1 – Waymouth's
MEM – minimum essential medium (Eagle's)
N-16 – Puck's et al.
NCTC-109 – Evans' et al.

I. BACKGROUND

A. Atherosclerosis and Atherogenesis

It is appropriate to introduce this text by defining atherosclerosis and atherogenesis. *Atherosclerosis* may be spoken of in clinical or in anatomical terms. Clinical signs and symptoms are either complications of anatomical alterations or are the direct results of advanced anatomical arterial lesions. *Atherogenesis* refers to the origin and evolution of anatomic alterations in the arterial wall.

The correlation of clinical symptomatology with anatomical alterations is by no means clear. Clinical disease can result from arterial stenosis, thrombosis or hemorrhage. Clinical symptoms may be due to arterial spasm. Extravascular factors may act as trigger mechanism.

Matters become more complicated when one attempts to identify and rank the factors which initiate or influence the progression of atherogenesis. Differences between species, races, ethnic groups, families, and individuals as to the incidence, degree, variety, and localization of lesions make the study of atherogenesis challenging. The world-wide distribution of atherosclerosis makes the study of atherogenesis imperative.

Many theories of atherogenesis have been proposed. Their credibility has been supported by experimental results or, at least, by the interpretation of results. None of the theories has gained universal acceptance. Some subscribe to a multifactorial concept. However, none of the proposed combinations of factors is applicable in every instance of atherogenesis. Others strive for simplification of the problem. However, every suggestion has ramifications. For example, hypercholesteremia, the most often singled-out factor, may be an individual's inborn characteristic, may result from an endocrinopathy, may come from renal disease, or may be of dietary origin. The blood cholesterol level may be out of the normal range as a result of liver disease, or may be influenced by bile flow, by intestinal evacuation, by climate, by exercise, etc. Free cholesterol, cholesteryl esters, and protein-bound cholesterol must be considered not only as part of the lipoid spectrum, but also in relation to non-lipoid blood constituents. Such is the downfall of oversimplification.

Inspired by the classical two-square diagram of Empedocles for the 4 seasons, 4 elements, and 4 sensations, POLLAK [1953b] devised sets of diagrams for atherogenic factors. The first diagram concerned 8 basic features: the artery—hereditary factors—blood factors—hemodynamic factors—lysis and clotting factors—neurovegetative factors—external factors—internal factors. Their interrelationships and interdependence were indicated by arrows.

By breaking up the 8 broad groups into more closely defined factors, one can construct 8 more diagrams. Further breakdown would lead to more and more diagrams. By splitting blood factors into lipoids, proteins, carbohydrates, etc., and then separating the components of the lipoid spectrum, one becomes aware that cholesterol is one of numerous atherogenic factors. The relative weight of each factor becomes important.

Many factors can be placed into several groups. Thus, wall thickness could be discussed as racial or genetically determined characteristic, or it could be treated under the heading of artery. Metabolic errors may be inborn or acquired, and may be manifested as blood factors or as arterial factors demonstrable by enzyme studies.

There is hardly a listing in a medical dictionary which has not been mentioned as an anatomical or functional etiologic factor or as a feature of atherogenesis. A detailed discussion of the etiology of atherogenesis would surely exceed the length of this monograph.

B. Research Avenues

Treatment of clinical atherosclerosis is becoming more and more successful. Of course, the ability to prevent clinical disease such as myocardial infarction would be preferable to the necessity of treating it. In the majority of instances—the magnitude of the majority is a point of conjecture—ischemic myocardial infarction and coronary artery thrombosis coincide. Therefore, major efforts have been exerted toward the lysis of blood clots and the prevention of thrombosis. The study of blood clotting has become a major research subject, especially since a number of clotting factors are also suspect as early atherogenic factors.

Clinical features of atherosclerosis and post-mortem examinations of arteries and receptor organs form the basis for epidemiologic studies. Observation of the terminal stages contributes little to the knowledge of early atherogenesis. Study of arteries separated from organs may lead to erroneous conclusions. Epidemiologic studies based solely on death certificates are misleading. One person dies *of* relatively moderate atherosclerosis, another person dies *with* but not of severe atherosclerosis. Epidemiologic studies are limited by the varying degrees of accuracy of diagnosis, by variable therapeutic successes, and by differing necropsy rates. Epidemiologists hope to find explanations for the uneven geographic distribution of clinical and anatomical atherosclerosis, for the diverse symptomatology, and for the variable extent, severity, and type of alterations among different ethnic groups. Correlations are sought with climate, race, body build, physical activity, dietary habits, and many more factors.

Comparative atherosclerosis is the study of atherogenesis in different species. Unintentional (spontaneous) atherosclerosis of reptiles, birds and mammals, in and out of captivity, is being scrutinized for common denominators and differences. The counterpart is intentional (experimental) atherosclerosis. Many attempts have been made to induce alterations in various species by manipulating one or more factors implicated as atherogenic, especially by controlling diets. For many years, the rabbit—the first animal in whom plaques were produced—was the only model for experimental atherogenesis. The rabbit has been joined or replaced by the rat, the dog, the pig, the chicken, the pigeon, and by the subhuman primates. Since it seems desirable to imitate the whole spectrum of human atherogenesis, the baboon—closest to the *homo sapiens*—seems best suited for experimental atherosclerosis.

Since the time when fatty plaques were first induced in cholesterol-fed rabbits, cholesterol has become a prime research target. Interest has grown with the biochemical observation that most patients with clinical atherosclerosis have a high blood cholesterol level. It has been further spurred by the findings of nutritionists that hypercholesteremia is a frequent characteristic of an overfed, affluent urban population. The simple formula—'high fat diet – hypercholesteremia – high incidence of atherosclerosis'—seems attractive. However, it has yet to be proven that atherogenesis in man can be prevented, arrested, or even slowed simply by a low-fat or low-cholesterol diet.

With the increasing sophistication of scientific thought and of research methods, the study of cholesterol was gradually replaced by the study of the whole lipoid spectrum. Interest shifted from the cholesterol/phospholipoid ratio to lipoprotein fractions, phospholipoids, and sterols. It had long been known to endocrinologists that the thyroid gland influences the blood cholesterol. The observation that the distribution of cholesteryl esters in various lipoprotein fractions differs for the female and the male was a new discovery. Study of the role of mono- and polyunsaturated fatty acids became popular. Attention began to be paid to the ratio between saturated and unsaturated fatty acids. Biochemical and physicochemical, clinical and epidemiologic researchers found a common interest. Nutrition-oriented epidemiologists claimed a higher incidence of atherosclerosis in countries where a diet rich in saturated fatty acids is consumed, than among ethnic groups whose diet contains a large proportion of unsaturated fatty acids.

While the study of blood lipoids has become intense, the study of other chemical components of the blood has been neglected. The statistically evident overlap between diabetes mellitus and atherosclerosis has not stimulated sufficient interest in the study of the carbohydrate metabolism in atherosclerosis. The only major efforts have been directed towards the control of diabetes as a means to retard atherogenesis. There is an apparent lack of interest on the part of investigators and granting agencies in the study of the protein metabolism within the frame of atherosclerosis research. The amino acid pattern of the protein moiety in lipoproteins may be as important as the pattern of cholesteryl esters of the lipoid moiety in lipoproteins.

The greater interest in lipoids than in other blood constituents may be ascribed to the fact that the atherosclerotic plaque contains large quantities of lipoids, especially cholesterol. The lipoid pattern of plaques reflects that of the patient's blood plasma. This finding lends support to the filtration theory of atherogenesis. However, there is solid evidence that both the normal and the atherosclerotic arterial walls are able to synthesize the components of the lipoid spectrum. Cholesterol synthesis by the artery and an exogenous cholesterol supply are parts of a homeostatic mechanism. The relative weights of internal and external factors are not constants. Internal factors are determined genetically, regulated hormonally, and depend on the general state of health of the body. External factors change with the forever changing environment.

Although the whole arterial system is exposed to the same blood, the distribution of atherosclerotic lesions throughout the system is uneven. There are inter- and intra-species differences. As a general rule, fatty patches are seen at the aortic cusps and near the ostia of the vertebral arteries of children; the most advanced lesions are seen in the abdominal aorta of adults. Some arteries feature only one type of lesion, the yellow streak. In other arteries different types of lesions and in different proportions are found.

Plaques do not develop synchronously. Atherogenesis is an episodic process. Explanations for these phenomena are sought by studying neurovegetative and hemodynamic factors. Many theories have been advanced, but none has universal validity.

Many investigators have become so involved in their particular areas of interest that they have lost sight of the substrate of the disease process—the artery itself. Some of the scientists who have contributed substantially to our understanding of atherogenesis, by constructing the pathways of cholesterol synthesis or by discovering the hormonal regulation of lipoprotein patterns, have never seen an artery. The study of the artery is at least as important as any other research in atherosclerosis.

The study of arteries in a living subject is technically difficult. *In vivo* cineangiography offers the best hope for quantitative evaluation of atherogenesis. The returns from stationary angiography and radiologic surveys have been meager. Occasionally, information about an arterial field has been gained during a surgical operation or on microscopic study of specimens removed by surgery.

Most studies of arteries are carried out through examination of necropsy material. Gross ranking of lesions is facilitated by post-mortem arteriography and by the preparation of resin or alloy casts of arteries. The correlation of anatomic findings with chemical studies and with clinical data is useful for the evaluation of dietary and pharmacologic management of atherosclerosis. Comparative studies of animal and human arteries by identical methods is another approach. Caution must be exercised in extrapolating to humans the observations made of animal arteries.

The intricate mechanisms of atherogenic initiation and progression can be investigated in many ways. Some aspects can be studied by light- and electronmicroscopy of arteries. Sample questions in this category are: What is the relative significance of the lumen/wall ratio? How important is the thickness of the intima-subintima, of the muscular layer, and of the total wall? What role does the intercellular pore play, with regard to plasma insudation, as compared with the cell membrane? Are anatomical alterations of the ground substance preceded by chemical alterations? Is the disturbance in acid mucopolysaccharides in the subendothelial layer a precursor, a concommitant phenomenon, or the sequel of structural alterations? Is the fat-laden cell which is typical of the yellow, fatty plaque a result of the transformation of an endothelial cell, a myocyte, a fibrocyte, a mast cell, or a blood cell? Could this cell derive from various cells? Do all fat-laden cells in a plaque have the same origin? Does this cell develop *in situ*, or does it migrate into the arterial intima from another site? How does a fibrous plaque develop? Can all fatty lesions undergo a change into a fibrous, pearly plaque? What factors determine the fate of a plaque, its stagnancy or growth, its progression into a combined lipoid-fibrous lesion, or into a pure fibrous lesion?

Other problems have to be answered by experimentation. Sample queries in this group are: What influences the cell membrane permeability? What is the role of anions and cations at the cell membrane and in the intercellular space? Are lipoids incorporated into cells by phagocytosis, pinocytosis, diffusion, or through lipfanogens? Can such process be enhanced, delayed, arrested or reversed and if so, by what means? Does the intravascular pressure, its height or oscillations, influence plasma insudation into the arterial wall? At what stage of atherogenesis does this become important? What is the interplay between intra- and extravascular pressure? The number of questions is endless. Each situation varies from one species to another, one subject to another, between arteries of different caliber, between arteries of the same caliber in different sites, and at different points along the course of an artery.

Some studies must be made *in vivo;* others may be made *in vitro*. Some can be made using vascular tissue cultures. *In vivo* observations provide guidelines for *in vitro* studies, and *vice versa*. Extrapolation, however, remains a serious problem.

II. EXTRACORPOREAL STUDIES

A. *Arterial Slices, Minces, Homogenates*

Extracorporeal studies of arteries include the gross, microscopic, and histochemical examination of vessels removed during surgical operation or at necropsy. They include chemical analysis of segments, slices, minces, homogenates, and extracts of arteries. Arterial tissues have been used for a variety of studies many of which are unrelated to atherosclerosis. Selected assays have been included in this text since some of the experiments could be adapted to vascular tissue cultures.

1. Ion Transport, Contractility

Epinephrine-induced contraction of rabbit aortic strips affects the influx and efflux of Ca^{45}, K^{42} and Na^{24}, according to BRIGGS and MELVIN [1961]. DANIEL [1965a, 1965b] followed the transport of Ca, Cl, K, Mg, CO_3, PO_4, SO_4, and glucose across the arterial cell membrane and the effect of sympathomimetic amines and of angiotensin on active ion transport and smooth muscle contractility. EHRENPREIS *et al.* [1965] used cholinesterase inhibitors, DANIEL and NASH [1965] used various diuretics, and MAXWELL *et al.* [1966] applied dl-norepinephrine-7-H^3. HCl and other compounds to influence contractility of rabbit aortic strips.

2. Diffusion Coefficients

KIRK and LAURSEN [1959] studied *in vitro* the diffusion of O_2, CO_2, lactate, glucose, and iodine in human aortic intima-subintima and media of subjects 10–39, 40–59, and 60–80 years. The diffusion coefficients increased with age, especially for substances of high molecular weight. Coefficients for atherosclerotic samples were about 70% higher than those for intact aortae. A significant relationship was found between lipoid content of aortic intima-subintima and the diffusion coefficient for lactate ($r = +0.53$, $t = 4.35$). The corresponding coefficient of correlation between tissue cholesterol and lactate diffusion was $+0.32$ ($t = 2.34$).

3. Respiration, Glycolysis

Aortae of rabbits, rats, human and other species—whole length or divided into 2 or 3 segments—have been used for respiration studies. Pieces being studied were either whole wall thickness or just the intima. Wet and dry tissues have been used for Warburg studies. Oxygen consumption of intact and of variously altered arteries are not the same. POLLAK [1968] pointed out that manifold experimental modifications and variances in expressing respiration rates and quotients make reconciliation of contradictory findings impossible. Glycolysis accounts for about 91% of glucose consumption by human aortic tissue, and respiration for the rest, the 2 processes supplying about equal caloric energy, according to FONTAINE *et al.* [1960].

4. Amino Acid Metabolism

According to HENRY [1963], rabbit aortae incorporate twice as much ^{14}C-leucine and ^{14}C-glycine as ^{14}C-prolin. KRISMAN and BAVINA [1954] found incorporation of ^{35}S-methionine, ^{14}C-glycine and ^{14}C-tyrosine significantly lower in rabbits' atherosclerotic aortae than in intact aortae.

5. Adenosine Triphosphate Synthesis

Studies of respiration quotients and of adenosine triphosphate (ATP) synthesis have been combined by SASAKI *et al.* [1965]. Incorporation of P^{32} into ATP by rat aortae and, to a lesser degree, the respiration of rat aortae decreased with aging. The oxygen consumption and ATP synthesis could be depressed by a magnesium-rich diet or enhanced by acetylcholine in the aortic tissues of young rats, but not in older animals.

6. Mucopolysaccharide Synthesis

PRIEST *et al.* [1960] observed that the incorporation of S^{35}-sulfate into mucopolysaccharides (MPS) of rat aortae could be reduced by estradiol. Utilization of C^{14}-glucose by rat aortae was reduced by estradiol, according to PRIEST and KOPLITZ [1962]. HASTINGS *et al.* [1968] found that the coronary arteries of swine synthesized significantly more MPS than the aortae or pulmonary arteries. They also found that estradiol reduced the uptake of S^{35}-sulfate by the coronary arteries of either sex, and increased uptake by the aortae of males but not of females. Testosterone reduced MPS synthesis by coronary arteries of male swine. These questions could be studied on the cellular level.

7. Cholesterol Synthesis

Many studies have been devoted to the ability of arteries to synthesize cholesterol. One can scan arteries from subjects who received radioactively labeled material during life, or one can measure the uptake of isotopes added to arterial tissues *in vitro*. The methodology of such experiments has often been modified for the sake of originality.

CHOBIAN [1968] recorded the incorporation of acetate-1-^{14}C and of mevalonate-2-^{14}C into cholesterol, cholestanol, and squalene by human arterial tissue. SIPERSTEIN *et al.* [1951], using stilbesterol, enhanced cholesterol synthesis by chicken and rabbit aortae. EISLEY and PRITHAM [1955] experimented successfully with minces of turkey aortae, and STEIN *et al.* [1963] with homogenates of rabbit aortae. LOFLAND *et al.* [1960] reported that cholesterol synthesis by aortic minces of a breed of pigeons susceptible to atherosclerosis was the same as that of a resistant breed.

8. Fatty Acid Synthesis

Rabbit aortic strips are capable of fatty acid synthesis, according to FELLER and HUFF [1955]. FOSTER and SIPERSTEIN [1960] found this to be true for the aortae of alloxan-diabetic rats. STEIN and STEIN [1962] reported that albumin has an inhibitory effect on fatty acid synthesis by aortic slices from baboons, dogs, rabbits, and rats.

9. Phospholipoid Synthesis

Phospholipoid synthesis by human aortae has been proven by ZILVERSMIT *et al.* [1961], with a significant increase of this process in atheromatous segments. NEWMAN *et al.* [1966] made analogous observations using normal and atheromatous aortae of rabbits. Qualitative and quantitative differences in the proportions of various phospholipoid fractions synthesized by beef and swine aortae and coronary arteries have been reported by NAKATANI *et al.* [1967a]. The influence of adrenalin and acetylcholine on the utilization of P^{32} by rat aortae has been studied by NAKATANI *et al.* [1967b].

Attempts to influence *in vitro* synthesis of ATP, MPS, cholesterol, fatty acids, and phospholipoids by estrogen, testosterone, epinephrine and other compounds, and through dietary manipulation have been made in various types of extracorporeal studies with arteries. Similar experiments have been applied to vascular tissue cultures.

10. Phospholipoid Synthesis by Macrophages

A report by DAY *et al.* [1966] deserves special attention since it represents a transition to vascular tissue culture work. 'Foam cells' from experimental aortic plaques of rabbits were isolated by incubation of the aortic intima in collagenase and elastase. These cells incorporated P^{32}-phosphate into lecithin and phosphatidyl inositol and, to a lesser extent, into phosphatidyl ethanolamine, sphingomyelin, and lysolecithin. The fat-laden cells separated from the aortic intima were not distinguishable from peritoneal macrophages. They are also indistinguishable from fat-laden macrophages identified by KASAI *et al.* [1964] in tissue cultures of experimental aortic lesions of rabbits.

B. Transmural Cholesterol Passage

Extracorporeal studies have been used to answer several important questions, such as the mode of transfer of cholesterol from the blood plasma into the arterial wall, and that concerning the unequal distribution of plaques in the arterial system. Another query has been directed to the gradient of cholesterol through the arterial wall.

1. Absorption, Adsorption

Innominate arteries of chicken were incubated by SIMMS [1936] and by SIMMS and STILLMAN [1937b] in a solution which contained the fat deposit-promoting serum 'B' factor (later renamed 'lipfanogens'). After 2 days incubation in serum ultrafiltrate and 4 days incubation in nutrient with serum lipfanogens, there was a considerable amount of fat present in the inner layers of the arterial wall.

HRŮZA *et al.* [1967] incubated thoracic aortae and collagen fibers from the tails of 6-week-old rats *in vitro* at 37°C for 24 hours in 1 to 2 ml of rat serum containing ^{14}C-cholesterol. There were no differences in the uptake of ^{14}C by aortae or by collagen fibers obtained from rats fed a basic diet and from rats fed an atherogenic diet for 11 weeks. The type of serum used for incubation was significant: Cholesterol uptake from the serum of old rats was smaller than uptake from the serum of young rats. Uptake by collagen fibers which had been artificially aged by incubation in 0.001% formaldehyde for 1 hour was greater than uptake of ^{14}C-cholesterol by untreated fibers. This nonphysiologic phenomenon could not be explained.

Discs 20 mm in diameter were punched out of pig aortae by BJORKSTEN [1952] and placed into a series of tanning agents for 15 seconds, 10 minutes, or for as long as 48 hours, then transferred to a carbon-colored cholesterol suspension for from 10 minutes to 16 hours. The adsorption and retention of cholesterol by the artificially aged aortae was ascribed to protein cross-linkage induced by the chemicals. Chromium sulfate was the most effective agent; cobalt sulfate, copper sulfate, and lead acetate were also effective. Attempts to induce release of the cholesterol were not successful.

2. Diffusion

To study cholesterol uptake at the endothelial level, JENSEN [1967a] dissected segments of the upper and lower thoracic aortae of rabbits and separated the intima-inner media from the outer media-adventitia. This permitted comparison of the central and the peripheral, traumatized part of cut-out samples. The samples were incubated in serum which had been labeled *in vivo* with 4-^{14}C-cholesterol. The uptake of the radioactive label by the edges of the samples was greater than by the central parts. Oxygen consumption was higher in the proximal part of the aortae than in the distal part. However, there was no difference in the conversion of glucose to lactic acid.

In another study, JENSEN [1967b] noted that there was a steep rise in the uptake of ^{14}C-cholesterol by rabbit aortae during the first 15 minutes of incubation. This phase was not temperature-dependent. He interpreted this as superficial cholesterol fixation to the endothelium. During the next, temperature-dependent phase there was a slow rise of the cholesterol curve. The transfer rate from serum to intima-media, and the resulting cholesterol concentration in the artery, paralleled the velocity of enzymatic reaction to substrate concentration.

Everted and noneverted rat aortae were compared by HASHIMOTO and DAYTON [1966]. Ligated everted aortae were incubated in a buffer with glucose, transferred to labeled serum, and later assayed for radioactivity. The noneverted aortae were filled with labeled serum, suspended in buffer, incubated, and later assayed. The ratio of unesterified to esterified cholesterol in 3 types of serum used was 100:0, 80:20, and 20:80, respectively. Three times as much unesterified cholesterol entered the aortae than esterified cholesterol. The results were interpreted as evidence of simple passive diffusion not requiring cellular activity.

3. Filtration, Pressure

WILENS [1951] ligated one end of human iliac arteries and introduced serum through the other end under an internal pressure regulated at 20 mm to 320 mm Hg. The rate of filtration reflected the pressure. The qualitative composition of the 24-hour filtrate was not dependent on the pressure or on the filtration period. However, the quantitative composition was time-dependent. The cholesterol in the filtrate was 20% to 50% lower than that of the serum. Up to 38% of the cholesterol was deposited in the intima. Albumin, globulin, and calcium were also retained in the arterial wall. To find the reason for the retention of these substances, WILENS and MCCLUSKEY [1952] expanded the experiments to include hemoglobin, egg albumin, phenolphthalein (which is eliminated by the kidneys) and Evans Blue (which is retained by the body). The retention of calcium was explained by its bondage to protein. The retention of cholesterol and proteins were ascribed to an inverse relation between molecular size and filtrability. Pressures ranging from 25 mm to 320 mm Hg were applied to iliac veins and to iliac arteries of the same subjects. At high pressure, the filtration rate through the thin-walled veins was 4 times faster than through the arteries. 20% of the serum cholesterol and 30% of the serum globulin passed through the artery; the corresponding percentages were 50 and 70 for the vein. The dializing properties were demonstrated by inserting a pipette filled with serum into the lumen of an artery or a vein suspended in saline solution and observing the rise of the fluid in the pipette. The osmotic effect of the nonfiltrable portion of serum lipoproteins was confirmed by reversing the arrangement, i.e. filling the pipette with 0.85% NaCl and suspending the blood vessels in serum.

4. Pulsation, Perfusion

Childrens' aortae and, because of their paucity of branches, adults' iliac arteries were selected by WILENS and MCCLUSKEY [1954] to study the permeability for cholesterol, phospholipoids, and total lipoids. They applied intermittent pulsation at 250/125 mm Hg at 40 pulses per minute. The pooled serum used for perfusion was replaced repeatedly to restore its initial condition, during the 2- to 3-day observation time. The filtrate contained 12.8% cholesterol, 13.2% phospholipoids, and 15.5% total lipoids, regardless of whether the serum was clear or chylous. Free and esterified cholesterol filtered through at comparable rates. Dilution of hypercholesteremic serum with physiologic saline accelerated the rate of lipoid deposit in the arteries. It was concluded that the process of lipoid entry into the arterial wall is not that of simple diffusion, but that it is pressure-dependent.

EVANS *et al.* [1956] used strips of human arteries, instead of whole vessels, in their studies of mechanical atherogenesis. Oxalated blood from patients with clinical atherosclerosis and from healthy young persons was pulsed against normal aortae from young adults at 80 pulses per minute. On the average, 185 bifringent particles per 100 microscopic fields were deposited within 72 hours pulsation with blood from patients with atherosclerosis. When blood from healthy persons was used, only 13.3 particles per 100 fields were counted. The presence of anisotropic particles in the arterial wall was correlated with the occurrence of clinical atherosclerosis. After perfusion with blood from healthy persons, non-cholesterol lipoids, but not cholesterol, could be identified in the arteries. The molecules were small enough to enter the intima and large enough to be trapped in the subintima. Results similar to those derived from the study of human arteries were obtained by EVANS *et al.* [1955] when rabbit aortae were perfused with pulsating serum.

The pulsation of lipemic plasma against chicken aortae at 60 pulses per minute and at 100 mm to 105 mm Hg pressure for 2 hours at 37°C resulted in the deposition of cholesterol and glycerides along arterial connective tissue fibers, between the elastic lamellae, but not in the musculature. Droplets smaller than 0.5 μ were identified in the intima, to a lesser degree in the inner media, and to a very slight degree in the outer media. This study by

GOLDBERG and MORANTZ [1957] confirmed the findings of others with regard to a gradient of deposited lipoids from the endothelium to the adventitia. The role of traumatization was confirmed by the observation that exposure of chicken arteries to α-toxin of *Clostridium Welchii* for 3 hours enhanced the deposit of lipoids.

The importance of the blood pressure for transmural passage of plasma through canine aortae was studied by DUNCAN and BUCK [1959] and by DUNCAN *et al.* [1959, 1962] in a combination of *in vivo* with *in vitro* experiments. Albumin was injected intravenously. The removed aortae were split into 3 layers. These were studied separately. The albumin entered the intima and left the adventitia at the same rate, i.e. at a constant gradient. Albumin concentration decreased in proportion to the decrease in flow rate. Along the length of the aortae, the flow correlated positively with the circumferential tension; it gradually decreased toward the distal end of the vessel.

In the next series of dogs, DUNCAN and BUCK [1961] submerged the aortae into 0.85% NaCl at 37° C and perfused them at 100 mm Hg with albumin-I^{135} labeled plasma for 3 hours. Transmural passage of albumin was faster than in the *in vivo* experiments. This was due to the equalizing of intramural and extramural pressures. Elevation of the blood pressure increased the entry rate of albumin into the ascending aorta. The increase was less into the upper thoracic and least into the lower thoracic aorta, making the gradient steeper. However, blood pressure itself was not considered an essential factor by DUNCAN *et al.* [1963], since its pulsatile nature could be excluded in the *in vitro* studies.

C. Organ Cultures

Studies of ion transport, contractility, or the respiration of arterial tissues, and studies of the transfer of cholesterol or albumin into the arterial wall, are based on short-term experiments with fresh material. For other studies, such as the investigation of the capability of arteries labeled *in vitro* to synthesize various compounds, it is essential to maintain the viability of blood vessels. Studies of arterial viability *in vitro* serve as a transition to vascular cultures.

1. Lipoid Synthesis

Aortae of several species were perfused with biologic fluids containing radioisotopes by WERTHESSEN [1961]. To simulate *in vivo* conditions and to assure viability of the tissues, the temperature and the pressure were controlled, the fluid was aerated, and the perfusate was replenished by glucose, amino acids, vitamins, etc. Aortae from young swine were used by SCHWENK and WERTHESSEN [1952], swine and beef aortae by WERTHESSEN *et al.* [1954], and calf aortae by WERTHESSEN *et al.* [1956], with similar results. Perfusion with 50% defibrinated blood, 50% White's solution and C^{14}-acetate resulted in active biosynthesis of cholesterol and other lipoids. There was a progressive quantitative increase in cholesterol from the origin of the aortae to the bifurcation. This difference was attributed to the uneven rate of glucose consumption by an aortic wall of uneven thickness. When glucose utilization was equal, about twice the amount of C^{14} was incorporated by calf aortae at 100 mm Hg as at 200 mm Hg in a 24-hour long experiment. In a 72-hour experiment, WERTHESSEN *et al.* [1955] found that synthesis by calf aortae was reduced if oxygen was absent.

A comparison was made between squalene and sterol synthesis by human renal, popliteal, and tibial arteries and by pigeon aortae. The vessels were perfused with buffered tissue culture nutrient by ST. CLAIR *et al.* [1968b]. All vessels were found capable of synthesizing squalene and sterols from dl-mevalonate-2-^{14}C. Two major fractions obtained by chromatography on alumina contained 99% of all lipoid radioactivity. For the pigeon, squalene synthesis correlated positively with the severity of atherosclerosis.

2. Lipoid Movements, Perfusate – Aorta – Perfusate

The movement of lipoids from the aorta into the blood was proven by NELSON and WERTHESSEN [1958]. Calf aortae and baboon aortae were first perfused for 2, 4, and 8 hours with 500 ml defibrinated blood labeled with 0.5 mc of l-C^{14}-acetate; then, after washing, they were perfused with unlabeled blood for from 6 to 24 hours. The baboon aortae released the radioactive label into the blood at a higher rate than the calf aortae. WERTHESSEN [1961] calculated the half-life of newly synthesized aortic cholesterol as 24 hours for the baboon and as 7 days for the calf aortae. The baboon aortae synthesized 35% to 45% cholesterol *in situ* and derived 55% to 65% from the blood plasma. From a 6-day perfusion system, 500 ml aliquots were saved and replaced at 24-hour intervals by fresh perfusate. To each portion, 0.09 mc of labeled acetate was added. After 2 days, there was a marked daily increment in C^{14} titre in the perfusate. Cholesterol released by the aortae was replaced by synthesized cholesterol. Homeostatic control of cholesterol movements was ascribed to hormones. Addition of paraaminobenzoic acid (PABA) caused a 55% increase in radioactivity counts of aortic lipoids, according to WERTHESSEN *et al.* [1956] and WERTHESSEN [1958, 1959]. PABA and nicotinic acid affected lipoid movements between calf aortae and perfusate. WERTHESSEN [1958, 1959, 1961] added estrone to the perfusate. There was no effect in the first 12 hours. Then, radioactive counts were 31×10^4 per minute, compared to 14×10^4 for control aortae perfused with no hormone additive. Testosterone and hydrocortisone also promoted incorporation of C^{14}.

MALINOW [1960] studied the effect of estradiol on chicken aortae, by combining short-term tissue cultures with chemical assays of tissue homogenates. Two isomers of estradiol enhanced, *in vitro*, the activity of a nonspecific alkaline phosphomonoesterase. Aortae were cut into 2 mm high rings and incubated for 72 hours in roller tubes containing balanced salt medium with 30% bovine serum, 0.05% ethanol, antibiotics, and 2 μg of either 17-α- or 17-β-estradiol. The alpha compound liberated 0.145 μM of phenol per mg of wet aortic tissues, and the beta compound liberated 0.136 μM. The corresponding controls, without hormones, liberated only 0.048 μM and 0.05 μM.

3. Lipoid Metabolism and Atherogenesis

Aortae of pigeons were perfused by LOFLAND *et al.* [1965] with Eagle's tissue culture medium labeled with acetate-l-^{14}C. Fatty acid synthesis was 5 to 6 times greater in atheromatous than in normal aortae. As the lesions became larger, a greater proportion of newly synthesized fatty acids was esterified with cholesterol. Perfusion with ^{14}C-carbon-l- or with ^{14}C-carbon-6-glucose resulted in a radioactive CO_2 production *via* hexose monophosphate about twice the magnitude of the CO_2 formed *via* glycolysis. LOFLAND and CLARKSON [1965] did not find this process related to the degree of atherogenesis. ST. CLAIR *et al.* [1968a] added acetate-l-^{14}C to the perfusate of aortae of White Carneau pigeons. No differences were found in the fatty acid composition of phospholipoids and glycerides between intact and atherosclerotic aortae. However, the cholesterol fraction of normal aortae contained 24.2% total fatty acids, whereas that of atherosclerotic aortae contained 61.9%.

Arterial perfusion with labeled cholesterol in serum has been combined with tissue culture studies by BAILEY [1964]. The thoracic aorta of the rabbit was tied over a 1 ml syringe through which 1 ml of rabbit serum with cholesterol-C^{14} was introduced. The aorta was kept in a culture medium at 30 mm Hg internal pressure, 95% O_2 and 5% CO_2 for 3 hours at 37°C. Upon washing, aortic strips were placed into nutrient with or without serum. Fresh aortae, prelabeled with cholesterol-C^{14}, were slit longitudinally, and each part cut into 3 horizontal segments. Pairs of segments were incubated in serum-free nutrient and in nutrient with 50% normal rabbit serum. In all experiments, the aortic label decreased when serum was added. Correspondingly, the label of the nutrient increased indicating excretion of cholesterol by the arterial wall into the medium. It was suggested that rabbit serum is relatively deficient in cholesterol-binding proteins.

Perfusion studies of lipoid synthesis were combined with studies of vascular viability by STRONG *et al.* [1957]. In nonperfused calf aortae, cellular details were lost within 72 hours. In perfused calf aortae, all the structures were preserved for up to 12 days *in vitro*. In the course of this study, the lag phase for deposit of sudanophilic material in the calf aortae was from 48 to 72 hours.

4. Viability of Blood Vessels

The introduction of arterial grafting stimulated interest in organ cultures of blood vessels. Since fresh donor arteries were not always available, it became important to determine the most efficient method of preserving the viability of arteries and the maximum length of time for which arteries could be preserved in a Vessel Bank. No attempt is made here to present a complete bibliography on this topic. References were selected which provide guidelines for vascular tissue culture work by answering such questions as to the course and speed of post-mortem degeneration of blood vessels.

PEIRCE *et al.* [1949] found that rapid freezing to 70°C or 72°C, storage in 100% autologous serum at 1°C to 4°C, and in Hanks' solution under helium were not suitable for preservation of aortae from adult man, young dogs, baboons and pigs. In Hanks' solution, and also in serum ultrafiltrate with 10% homologous serum at 1°C to 4°C, aortae of these species remained viable for 14 days. LAZZARINI [1952] applied the same methods to various arteries and to veins of man, with comparable results. SWAN *et al.* [1952] rapidly froze canine aortae in a nutrient with CO_2 and alcohol, and subsequently stored them in a frozen state. Such aortae were as suitable for grafting after 25 days' storage as were fresh aortae. For grafting, aortae of dogs younger than 2 years were superior to aortae from older dogs.

Criteria for the selection of human aortae for homografts were established by DETERLING *et al.* [1953] on the basis of organ culture results. Body temperature at death, the cause and mode of death, and freedom from bacteria were held important. Alkaline phosphatase began to disappear 2 hours after death, glycogen after 48 hours, and mucopolysaccharides after 96 hours. The longer the time between death and refrigeration of an artery, the poorer the tissue culture results. A 4-hour post-mortem period was found to be critical for tissue viability.

PEIRCE *et al.* [1949, 1952] checked the viability of arteries by silver impregnation of endothelial surface preparations. LAZZARINI [1952] examined the tissues histologically. BELLMAN *et al.* [1956] monitored the viability of dog aortae by combined isotope and respiration studies. In the latter study, aortae were put into a balanced salt solution with 10% of homologous serum and antibiotics at 2°C to 6°C and incubated for 4 hours in Krebs-Ringer bicarbonate solution with 1 mc carrier-free S^{35}-sodium sulfate per 100 ml. There was progressive decrease of S^{35} incorporation. After 1 week, the decrease was 10% to 20%; yet, after 4 weeks' storage, the zero point had not been reached. Oxygen consumption by the arteries paralleled S^{35} incorporation.

5. Synthetic Grafts

As stored arterial segments were replaced by synthetic material for grafting by surgeons, interests of tissue culture workers shifted from arteries to artificial prosthetic material. It became fashionable to combine *in vivo* and *in vitro* studies.

MACKENZIE and LOEWENTHAL [1960] studied crimpled nylon grafts removed from human hosts 'en face'. The grafts were coated by an endothelial cell layer. This finding agreed with a dozen reports published during the preceding decade. The terms 'neointima' and 'pseudointima' were applied to the cell sheets which developed on synthetic material. It was believed that the endothelial cells originated in the host artery at both ends of the graft. STUMP *et al.* [1962] kept dacron prostheses in place in canine aortae for 3 years. Upon silver impregnation of 'en face' preparations nuclei could not be visualized. However, in stained pellicle (Häutchen) preparations endothelial cells with nuclei were identifiable. LAZZARINI [1959] obtained comparable results with 6- to 12-week-old dacron grafts from man, dog and rabbit. ROBERTSON [1965a] found the neointima smooth, but the pseudointimal endothelial cells growing in a disorderly fashion and growing slower than normal cells.

PARSHLEY *et al.* [1950] noted many 'round cells' with fat globules in grafts removed from canine aortae. LAZZARINI [1961b, 1961c] found that atherosclerotic alterations developed faster in grafts than in host arteries. The neointima of homografts in man and in 6- to 13-month-old dogs reacted similarly to atherosclerotic human arteries with regard to uptake of labeled cholesterol, according to LAZZARINI [1962b, 1962c].

The sequence of the experiments cited above was from *in vivo* to *in vitro*. The opposite approach was used by FABRIZIO [1961]. A layer of fibroblasts was developed using tendon sheets of mongrel dogs in *in vitro* cultures on fragments of dacron. The cell-coated material was used as a substitute 'biologic membrane' and implanted into donor dogs as the leaflet of a heart valve. There was no rejection of this autologous transplant, and no further cell growth occurred on the implanted dacron valve.

6. Dacron Hubs

The growth of cells on the surface of synthetic grafts could be referred to as a type of '*in vivo* cell culture'. STUMP *et al.* [1963] implanted knitted, crimpled DeBakey dacron prostheses, 5 cm long and 2 cm in diameter, into the thoracic aortae of young pigs. A dacron hub, 0.5 cm^2 in diameter and 0.2 cm thick, was suspended within the prosthesis by smooth polyethylene sutures. Both the hub and the prosthesis were removed after periods ranging from 1 to 42 days. After 7 days, the hub was covered with endothelial cells. After 14 days, hub and prosthesis were coated with cells. The sutures were without cells after 20 or 21 days. A coagulum of erythrocytes, monocytes, and up to 4 layers of endothelial cells were found, and fat-laden mononuclear cells. Foreign-body giant cells were seen above fibroblasts, smooth muscle cells, and collagen after a 25 to 42 day observation period. O'NEAL *et al.* [1964], using young pigs and adult dogs, suspended dacron hubs in aortae without prostheses. The hubs were removed from the pigs' aortae 8 to 28 days after implantation; in the dog aortae the hubs were left in place for up to 170 days. Pellicle, en face, and histologic examinations were supplemented by electron microscope studies to identify endothelial cells, fibroblasts, and smooth muscle cells on the surface of the hubs.

The conclusion that the endothelial cells, and possibly also the other types of cells, derive from circulating blood cells must be seriously questioned. It is known that normal endothelial cells and fat-laden cells can become detached from the vascular intima, circulate in the blood stream, cause cell emboli, seed themselves at remote sites and, at least in the case of endothelial cells, proliferate at a new site. Most likely, the trauma to the host artery when the hub is inserted provides sufficient impetus to cell detachment.

7. Pulsating Tubes

Latex tubes and distensible plastic tubes, sealed at both ends, were implanted subcutaneously in rats and guinea pigs by GLAGOV *et al.* [1968a, 1968b]. The diameter and pulsation of the tubes were regulated by a pump. Water was pumped through the tubes at 60 to 180 pulses per minute. In one weeks' time, the tubes became coated with fibroblasts and with cells which resembled human fetal smooth muscle cells, and with collagen. There was much less of a reaction, and little alignment of cells, along nonpulsating tubes.

III. NON-VASCULAR TISSUE CULTURES

The logical sequence of this text would be to proceed from vascular organ cultures to vascular tissue and cell cultures. However, a place had to be found for nonvascular cultures. Essays dealing with the formation of capillaries in nonvascular tissue explants are of interest because they refer to vascular endothelial cells. Essays dealing with lipoid metabolism of nonvascular cells in tissue culture—though only remotely related to the problems of atherogenesis—are important because many of these experiments have also been carried out with vascular cells. The references which have been selected should serve as starting points for further studies.

1. Growth of Capillaries in Tissue Explants

Capillaries without blood cells were noted by RIENHOFF [1922] in *in vitro* cultures of meso- and meta-nephros of 8- to 10-day-old chick embryos. LEWIS [1931] saw new capillaries containing degenerated erythrocytes in 700 of 2,000 cultures of 7- to 8-day-old chick embryo organs. SCRIBA [1935] made similar observations in 25% to 30% of limb bud cultures of 9-day-old chick embryos, and TÖRÖ [1937] confirmed these findings using chick embryo lungs and mesonephros. MURRAY and STOUT [1944] described endothelial cells in capillaries in a 6-day-old culture of the rib of a 20-day-old rat fetus. Vascular channels with blood cells and forming an anastomosing network were seen in cultures of liver explants in 1- to 3½-month-old human embryos by BENEWOLENSKAJA [1929]. WHITE and PARSHLEY [1951] found that a capillary network developed in 86.8% of 38 cultures of the bone marrow of adult chickens. Red and white blood cells were seen in these capillaries after 23 and 28 days, respectively.

CAMERON and CHAMBERS [1937] identified endothelial cells in tissue cultures of a congenital human angioma, and MURRAY and STOUT [1944] described vascular channels lined by endothelial cells in cultures of a human adult hemangioendothelioma. The culture of a rib metastasis of human angiosarcoma yielded endothelial cells for COMAN [1942].

Endothelial cells were also seen by Maximow [1925] in cultures of pia mater. He thought that they originated from the arteries of the explant. The cells were described as having a transparent cytoplasm and a pale nucleus, with a short life span, and not capable of phagocytosis of carmine particles. The pia mater, choroid plexus, vena portae and vena cava of rabbits were studied in tissue cultures by Silberberg [1929], and 'endothelial cells' were seen 24 hours after inoculation. However, the description of these cells matches all the characteristics of fibroblasts. Herzog and Schopper [1931] grew endothelial cells from capillaries of the pia-arachnoid of guinea pigs in 3- to 4-day-old cultures.

2. Lipoid Uptake from Nutrient

A number of recent references to lipoid metabolism of nonvascular cells *in vitro* have been selected for discussion here to suggest new projects to vascular tissue culture workers.

Cultures of mouse lymphoblasts of the BM III strain and cultures of fibroblasts of the L-strain were treated by Bailey [1964] with cholesterol suspension in Tween 80 and with radioactively labeled cholesterol in albumin. Bailey [1964, 1965] found that cholesterol continuously enters cells, and that cholesterol synthesized from mevalonic acid-C^{14} is continuously excreted from the cells, probably combined with certain serum α-globulins. Glucose and acetate were the main sources of lipoid synthesis. Bailey [1966] noted that addition of serum, or of serum lipoids, decreased lipoid synthesis. The suppression of the uptake of acetate-^{14}C into lipoids upon the addition of serum was confirmed by Geyer [1967] in studies with HeLa cells.

Rothblat *et al.* [1966, 1967] found that the uptake of 4-^{14}C-cholesterol by mouse leukemia lymphoblasts (L-5178Y) was directly related to serum cholesterol concentration. In their experiments, cells were grown in the presence of 1-^{14}C-acetate for 18 hours, washed, suspended in a buffer, and exposed to 10% horse serum with 7-α-(^{3}H)-cholesterol. Exogenous ^{3}H-cholesterol was incorporated, while cells with ^{14}C-cholesterol lost none of their radioactivity. It was concluded that endogenous cholesterol, whether derived by uptake or by synthesis *de novo*, does not change places with the cholesterol present in the nutrient. Moskowitz [1967] found that fatty acids induced steatosis of L-fibroblasts and of rabbits' liver cells, commensurate with rising acidosis of the nutrient. Bailey [1967] stated that, of all the lipoid, triglycerides were utilized best, while cholesterol was used least. HARARY *et al.* [1967] noted that linoleic acid, and also arachidonic acid, promoted the growth of HeLa cells and rat heart cells; palmitate did not. However, according to BAILEY [1961], neither linoleic acid nor stearic acid had any effect on the cholesterol content of mouse BM III lymphoblasts. ROTHBLAT and KRITCHEVSKY [1968] reviewed the bulk of references to cholesterol metabolism of nonvascular cells in tissue culture.

3. Lipoid Uptake from Added Serum

Mouse lymphoblasts BM III were exposed by BAILEY [1961] to human adult serum containing 218.7 mg cholesterol per 100 ml, resulting in cells containing 3.7% cholesterol. On exposure to human cord blood with 97 mg cholesterol per 100 ml, the cell cholesterol was 2.25%. Exposure of the cells to rabbit serum with 85 mg cholesterol per 100 ml resulted in a cell cholesterol content of 7.8%. The conclusion—that the serum cholesterol level is not a decisive factor in cholesterol uptake by cells—was revised by BAILEY *et al.* [1961] due to the results of further experiments in which BM III cells were exposed to serum of patients with or without atherosclerosis. The average serum cholesterol of the first group was 13.6% higher than that of the latter group. After 4-day exposure, cells grown with hypercholesteremic serum contained 13.6% more cholesterol than cells grown with control serum. Cells grown with rabbit serum which contained 2,148 mg cholesterol per 100 ml and cells grown with normal rabbit serum which had 85.8 mg cholesterol per 100 ml, contained 22.25% and 7.8% cholesterol, respectively. The authors concluded that there is no experimental evidence which would suggest that factors other than hypercholesteremia influence the cholesterol content of cells.

L-929 mouse fibroblasts were exposed to normo- and hypercholesteremic swine serum by CHOI *et al.* [1968]. Neither type of serum had any influence on the cell proliferation of primary cultures. Cell counts of subcultures exposed to hypercholesteremic serum were 50% lower than cell counts of controls. Cell death was more rapid under the influence of hypercholesteremic serum. The rate of ^{3}H-thymidine, ^{14}C-leucine, and ^{14}C-glycine incorporation of surviving cells was not impaired by the hypercholesteremic serum. The reaction of the 'cell lines' from the intima-media of swine aortae to normo- and hypercholesteremic swine serum was the same as that of L-929 mouse cells.

The growth stimulating effect of chondroitinsulfate A (CS-A), C (CS-C), keratosulfate, and phospholipoids on HeLa cells was studied by MORRISON *et al.* [1965a]. All substances promoted cell growth, as determined by cytocrit, by hemocytometer counts, and by the dry weight of cells. MORRISON *et al.* [1965b] treated cultures of mouse L-cells, HeLa cells, and human amnion cells for 72 hours with human hyperlipemic serum. To 100 ml of nutrient, 1 mg of CS-A was added for from 3 to 48 hours; before trypsinization, 100 μg^{32} P were introduced. CS-A had no effect on HeLa cells after 3-hour exposure, but after 6 hours the dry weight of the cells and the amount of ribonucleic acid increased and P^{32} uptake by phospholipoids doubled. After 5-hour exposure, CS-A increased RNA and DNA of mouse L-cells. The passage of P^{32} into phospholipoids of mouse L-cells and human amnion cells was increased after 24-hour exposure to CS-A. After exposure to human hyperlipemic serum, the growth of mouse L-cells was inhibited. The growth of human amnion cells and P^{32} uptake was retarded.

Metabolic studies of nonvascular cells are favored by investigators and granting agencies. Nevertheless, they have limited value in atherosclerosis research. In the above cited studies, mouse L-fibroblasts of several strains, mouse lymphoblasts MB III and L-5178Y, and the classical HeLa cells were used most often; further rabbit liver cells, rat heart cells and human amnion cells. The extrapolation of experimental results from these cells to human arterial cell behavior should be made with restrain, if at all.

The fibroblast, whether from mouse or man, is the cell least suited to the study of lipoid metabolism. LAZZARINI [1959, 1961b, 1962a, 1962d] demonstrated that human and canine aortic endothelial cells are far more active than aortic fibroblasts. Fibroblasts from 22 different parts of the chick embryo were studied by PARKER [1933], and 5 strains with different culture characteristics were identified from them. Aortic fibroblasts had the lowest energy. WHITE and PARSHLEY [1951] noted that the lag phase for chicken aortic fibroblasts was longer than that for fibroblasts from other sites. CASTOR *et al.* [1952] compared 13 primary cell lines of fibroblasts from different anatomic sites and 3 permanent cell lines. Differences were recorded with regard to proliferation rate, MPS production rate, and the quantity of anthrone-positive material. KASAI and POLLAK [1964a] reported that aortic fibroblasts and tendon fibroblasts of the same rabbit differed morphologically. POLLAK and ADACHI [1968] demonstrated that rabbit aortic and tendon fibroblasts differed from each other more than rabbit aortic fibroblasts differed from human aortic fibroblasts. Human atheroma cells differ metabolically from human xanthoma cells, according to ROBERTSON [1968b,

1969]. In the light of such information, the studies comparing cells of entirely different anatomic origin, and differing species, should be reevaluated. To those studying atherogenesis, the role of the endothelial cell and the smooth muscle cell with regard to lipoid metabolism is of greater interest than the role of the fibroblast.

According to LAZZARINI [1963d], one of the most important factors in comparative studies is the length of time for which cells are exposed to an environment. BAILEY [1961] concluded that in the ultimate analysis lipoid metabolism is related to the cell type. It should be added that, when speaking of the 'cell type', one should bear in mind 3 fundamental features: (a) the 'type' itself, (b) the anatomic origin of the cell, and (c) its origin by species.

IV. VASCULAR TISSUE CULTURES

A. Introduction

Keeping all the limitations of tissue culture work in mind, it may be safely stated that this young discipline can be profitably applied to the study of atherogenesis on the cellular level, especially of its early stages.

There are many bridges between organ, tissue and cell cultures. One can start a culture by placing a whole organ—a blood vessel—into a nutrient. One can utilize a part of a vessel—for example, with the intima-media separated from the outer layers—to start a tissue culture. One can start a cell culture with cells separated from the vessel wall, or with cells isolated from a tissue culture and transferred to a subculture. The latter can be pursued by removing the explant after the outgrowth of cells and by following the fate of the remaining cells, or it can be accomplished by removing cells from the primary culture and transferring them to a secondary culture. The term 'vascular tissue culture' is used broadly, embracing organ, tissue, and cell cultures.

One should always look at a blood vessel as part of the whole body, and at each artery as part of the receptor organ. Coronary arteries are part of the heart and renal arteries are part of the kidneys. For tissue culture work, vessels must be separated from organs. The term 'cardiovascular tissue culture' refers to heart and blood vessels. In this text, reference to cardiac cultures is made only rarely, where a comparison has previously been made between cultures of myocardial and arterial cells. The bibliography pertaining to vascular tissue and cell cultures is being reviewed exhaustively, critically, and, hopefully, constructively (up to June 1969).

B. Historical Notes

The tissue culture was introduced by Harrison [1910]. The 1st report on vascular tissue cultures was made by Carrel and Burrows [1910]. They observed very delicate, palm-like cells 3 days after inoculating autologous plasma with arteries of adult dogs and cats. The vegetation was weak, and growth stopped entirely within a few days. The next report, made by BLOOM [1929], concerned the growth of fibroblasts in 15- to 17-day-old cultures of aortic explants from guinea pig embryos. The 3rd report was more elaborate. SHIBUYA [1931] grew endothelial cells from adult rabbit aortae within 24 to 48 hours after planting. The cells lived for 6 to 12 days. The appearance of fibroblasts and histiocytes in 6-day-old cultures was interpreted as the metamorphosis of endothelial cells into other cell types.

Reports on endothelial cells and on the formation of capillaries in tissue cultures of the pia mater were made by MAXIMOW [1925], SILBERBERG [1929] and by HERZOG and SCHOPPER [1931].

While studying the viability of arteries for homotransplants, PEIRCE *et al.* [1949], PARSHLEY *et al.* [1950], and DETERLING *et al.* [1953] contributed valuable information concerning optimal times for obtaining, handling, and storing arteries. PARSHLEY *et al.* [1953] continued with a thorough description of the various cell types grown in cultures of arteries from several species.

None of these studies were made under the flag of atherosclerosis research. SIMMS [1936] cultured chicken aortic cells, and SIMMS and STILLMAN [1937a and on[1]] identified several serum factors which affect the growth of aortic fibroblasts. Later, SIMMS *et al.* [1947 and on] discovered that lipoid transport on the cellular level is regulated by the ratio of lipfanogens to antilipfanogen. A bridge to atherosclerosis research by cell culture was thus established.

LAZZARINI [1959] observed the development of atherosclerotic alterations in homografts removed from dog and man. This led to research in atherosclerosis, utilizing vascular tissue cultures. He made the study of the effect of lipoid emulsions on arterial intimal cells in tissue culture in relation to atherosclerosis the theme of a thesis. The numerous references listed under LAZZARINI [1952-1960b], LAZZARINI-ROBERTSON [1961a–1968], and ROBERTSON [1965a and on[1]] attest to his contributions in the field of vascular tissue cultures.

Another stimulus came from RUTSTEIN *et al.* [1958] who used human aortic and myocardial cell cultures. They discussed the protective effect of linoleic acid and the lipoidosis-enhancing effect of stearic acid on the basis of study of these acids in the course of induced lipoid deposition in human aortic cell cultures. Although the observations were later found to be incorrect by RUTSTEIN *et al.* [1964], the original report had a marked impact on vascular and nonvascular tissue culture work.

[1] 'And on' used instead of listing all subsequent references.

Another group began work in the field of vascular tissue cultures in 1960. KOKUBU and POLLAK [1961 and on], KOIDE and POLLAK [1963 and on], and KASAI and POLLAK [1964 and on] compared aortic cultures from normo- and hypercholesteremic rabbits, identified step-by-step the 4 cell types which can be grown from arteries, studied the effect of nicotine and cigarette smoke. The contributions of this research group may be seen from the bibliography.

BRANWOOD [1961a, 1963] summarized his results with human arterial cells in his text on the pathogenesis of coronary atherosclerosis. A large series of reports has been contributed by MORRISON *et al.* [1963 and on] and by MURATA *et al.* [1965 and on]. They studied the effect of mucopolysaccharides, alone or combined with lipoid, on the growth and the metabolism of chicken aortic cells.

One of the landmarks of the first decade of atherosclerosis research on the cellular level was the Cardiovascular Tissue Culture Conference held at Dover, Delaware (USA), May 25–26, 1961. All the active research teams were represented, as recorded by BRANWOOD [1961b]. Financial support for the meeting and publication of discussions had been refused by experts who thought that all the questions which could possibly be answered by vascular tissue culture work had already been answered. In taking issue with this misconception, POLLAK [1963] cited his lecture at the International Cardiology Colloquium in Brussels (May 22–25, 1962), entitled 'Elucidation of atherogenesis by cardiovascular cell culture',—an endless chain of questions interrupted by sporadic answers. And in another lecture on 'Tissue cultures in atherosclerosis', presented at the Third Interamerican Congress on Atherosclerosis in Buenos Aires (April 28–May 4, 1968), POLLAK [1969] stated that although many of the questions posed years ago had been answered, the chain of questions was not getting any shorter. Every answer has created new questions.

C. Methodology

In any research field, the approach to a problem is crucial to the outcome of the experiment. This is certainly true of vascular tissue cultures. The choice of explant and nutrient, of the culture environment, even the choice of glassware, influence the results. It is not simple to reconcile divergent reports.

The main reason for the meager harvest of cells by early investigators lies in the culture technic. This is true of the work with pia-arachnoid and of the work with arteries, as well.

Table I. Selection of explants by species and by anatomic site

Species	Source	Intact	Altered	References, footnotes
Cat	aorta	+		CARREL and BURROWS, 1910[1]; PARSHLEY *et al.*, 1953
Chicken	aorta	+		SHIBUYA, 1931[2]; SIMMS, 1936, 1951; SIMMS and HARMISON, 1966; SIMMS and SANDERS, 1942; SIMMS and STILLMAN, 1937a, 1937c, 1937d, 1937e; SIMMS *et al.*, 1947[1], 1954, 1956; LAZZARINI, 1955, 1959[3], 1961b[4]; FREEMAN and MORRISON, 1961; MORRISON *et al.*, 1963; MURATA, 1968; MURATA *et al.*, 1965, 1966, 1967a, 1967b
Dog	aorta	+		CARREL and BURROWS, 1910[1]; SIMMS and STILLMAN, 1937d, PEIRCE *et al.*, 1949; PARSHLEY *et al.*, 1950, 1953; PARSHLEY and DETERLING, 1953; LAZZARINI, 1959, 1961a; 1961e, 1962d, 1963a; CURTIS and GALVIN, 1963; ROBERTSON, 1967a
			+	LAZZARINI, 1961b[5]
	carotid	+		PARSHLEY *et al.*, 1953
Guinea	aorta	+		BLOOM, 1929; PARSHLEY *et al.*, 1953
Goat	aorta	+		PARSHLEY *et al.*, 1953
Man	aorta	+		PEIRCE *et al.*, 1949; PARSHLEY *et al.*, 1953[6]; LAZZARINI, 1955, 1959, 1960a, 1962c[7], 1962e; INGENITO *et al.*, 1958; RUTSTEIN *et al.*, 1958, 1964; BRANWOOD, 1961a, 1963[8]
		+	+	LAZZARINI, 1961a, 1961b, 1961d, 1961e, 1963a; BEHBEHANI *et al.*, 1965; ROBERTSON, 1965a, 1965b, 1967a, 1967b, 1968a, 1968b, 1969; POLLAK and ADACHI, 1968
	coronary	+	+	LAZZARINI, 1960a, 1960b[9], 1961b, 1962b, 1962d, 1962e[9]; BRANWOOD, 1961a, 1963
	femoral	+		POLLAK *et al.*, 1962a; BRANWOOD, 1963; POLLAK and BURNS, 1965
		+	+	POLLAK and ADACHI, 1968
	iliac	+	+	LAZZARINI, 1961b, 1962b, 1962d, 1962e[9]
	mesenteric	+	+	LAZZARINI, 1961b, 1962b, 1962d, 1962e[9]
	popliteal	+	+	POLLAK and ADACHI, 1968
	pulmonary	+		POLLAK and ADACHI, 1968
	subclavian	+		PARSHLEY *et al.*, 1953; LAZZARINI, 1961b, 1962b, 1962d, 1962e[9]
	tibial	+	+	POLLAK and ADACHI, 1968
Minipig	aorta	+		CHOI *et al.*, 1968; FLORENTIN *et al.*, 1968, 1969

Table I. (Continuation)

Species	Source	Intact	Altered	References, footnotes
Monkey	aorta	+		PARSHLEY *et al.*, 1953; ROBERTSON, 1965a
Mouse	aorta	+		LAZZARINI, 1959
Pig	aorta	+		LAZZARINI, 1963a; ROBERTSON, 1965a, 1967a
Pigeon	aorta	+		SMITH *et al.*, 1965[10]
Rabbit	aorta	+		SHIBUYA, 1931[1,2]; PARSHLEY *et al.*, 1953; LAZZARINI, 1959; LAZZARINI and WEISSMANN, 1960; KOKUBU and POLLAK, 1960, 1961a
		+	+	ENGEL, 1961; ENGEL and POLLAK, 1961; KOKUBU, 1961; KOKUBU and POLLAK, 1961b, 1961c; KOKUBU *et al.*, 1961; KOIDE and POLLAK, 1962, 1963a, 1963b, KOIDE *et al.*, 1963; KASAI and POLLAK, 1964a, 1964b; KASAI *et al.*, 1964; POLLAK, 1961, 1963, 1967, 1968, 1969; POLLAK and ADACHI, 1968; POLLAK and BURNS, 1965; POLLAK and KOKUBU, 1961; POLLAK and KASAI, 1963, 1964; POLLAK and WADA, 1966, 1967, 1968a, 1968c; WADA and POLLAK, 1966, 1967, 1968a, 1968c; POLLAK *et al.*, 1960, 1962a, 1962b
	coronary	+		LAZZARINI, 1959
Rat	aorta	+		AYKAN, 1964; PRIEST *et al.*, 1960; PRIEST and PRIEST, 1964
		+	+	WEXLER and THOMAS, 1967[11]
	carotid	+		WEXLER and THOMAS, 1967
Rhesus	aorta	+		RUTSTEIN *et al.*, 1964; MURATA, 1968; KAO *et al.*, 1968[12]
Sheep	aorta	+		SIMMS and STILLMAN, 1937d

[1] Adult, [2] embryo, [3] 19 day embryo, [4] 1 week old, [5] experimental atherosclerosis, [6] under 45 years, [7] under 30 years, [8] intima, [9] 6 to 78 years, [10] 2 breeds, [11] fibrous lesions, [12] media.

1. The Explant

The choice of the anatomical site for a vascular explant is most important. It may make scant difference which muscle one selects for a culture, or which part of a normal liver. It makes quite a difference whether one cultures an artery or a vein, a large artery or a small one, a thick-walled or a thin-walled artery. Comparable arteries from several species do not yield the same results. The donor's age may make a difference. Two segments of the same artery may differ. One cannot expect the same results from culturing an intact and an atherosclerotic artery. Atherosclerotic lesions of varying type lead to dissimilar results.

a) Selection by Site

The aorta has been used as a source for vascular culture far more often than other arteries. Veins have been used seldom—at least, results of cultures of cells from veins have not been reported. Most investigators have worked with intact arteries. Some have worked with aortae and smaller arteries with spontaneous or experimental lesions. Members of many species have been used as donors for explants (table I). Gaps in the available list should be filled in the future. The list should be expanded in all its ramifications.

b) Preparation of Explants

Tissues removed from the living or the deceased can be planted immediately, or they can be planted after storage. Usually, the blood vessel is rinsed in an isotonic salt solution before it is dissected. SHIBUYA [1931] placed rabbit aortae into Ringer's solution; PARSHLEY *et al.* [1953] used NaCl solution or nutrient for segments of dog aortae, at 4°C. PARSHLEY and DETERLING [1953] placed dog aortae into Simms' X6 solution or into 10% serum, at 4°C. LAZZARINI [1959] and POLLAK [1961] transferred tissues to Hanks' solution during the preparation of explants for culture.

SIMMS and STILLMAN [1937c, 1937d, 1937e] kept chicken aortae in Tyrode solution at 4°C up to 4 days. Simms' X6 solution plus serum ultrafiltrate was used for storage by SIMMS and SANDERS [1942], SIMMS [1951], SIMMS *et al.* [1954, 1956], and SIMMS and HARMISON [1966]. PEIRCE *et al.* [1949] stored aortae of baboons, dogs, pigs, and men in Hanks' solution with 10% of homologous serum. PARSHLEY *et al.* [1950] and PARSHLEY and DETERLING [1953] experimented with dog aortae. Comparison of cultures after 10-day storage at 4°C with cultures of fresh aortae pointed clearly to the superiority of fresh material. MORRISON *et al.* [1963] and MURATA *et al.* [1966, 1967] placed chicken aortae into 1% trypsin overnight at 20°C before planting.

c) Choice of Explants

Culture results vary with the type of explants. BRANWOOD [1961a, 1963] used a pellicle (Häutchen) of intimal endothelial cells separated from the artery. Such preparations yielded a less varied cell population than did whole-wall-thickness explants. KAO *et al.* [1968] cultured 2 mm discs of Rhesus aortic media to obtain cultures of smooth muscle cells.

The intima with endothelial cells attaches to the support when one places an explant on the support face-down. If such explant is removed early, endothelial cells will prevail. Fibroblasts will predominate if the explant is placed with the adventitia facing the support. ROBERTSON [1967a, 1967b] prepared a 'sandwich' or 'envelope' by placing the explant between 2 cover slips so that the intima faced one cover slip and the adventitia the other.

From a ring-shaped segment placed onto a flat surface, intimal cells grow into the lumen and adventitial cells grow from the outer surface. HERZOG and SCHOPPER [1931] everted such rings so that the adventitia faced the lumen. Much of the adventitial growth is removed at the time the explant is removed with the plasma clot. The cells which grew from the intima are left behind. This method has been used extensively by LAZZARINI [1959 and on] and by POLLAK [1960 and on].

A solid support is needed when a monolayer culture is desired. The wall of a flask or test tube or a cover slip provides this support. Control over the cell population will be lost if the explant is placed into liquid nutrient. Clearly, the choice of procedure depends on the aims of the investigator.

d) *Removal of Explants*

The first outgrowth of cells may be seen as early as 24 hours after planting. Since fibroblasts appear on the 5th or 6th day, propagate rapidly and displace other cells, the explant has to be removed as soon as the first cells have appeared if one wants to isolate endothelial cells. If one desires a complete spectrum of vascular cells, the explant should be left *in situ*. KASAI and POLLAK [1964] fixed the appearance of smooth muscle cells as the 12th day after planting. In most instances these cells were not seen before the 16th or 17th day. Because of early explant removal, myocytes have rarely been seen.

The composition of the cell population in primary culture changes constantly. The various cell types grown from blood vessels differ as to their lag phase, growth curves, and longevity. Different cells have different nutritional requirements. Their growth curves are not parallel. The aging of cells has to be considered in studies of respiration and metabolism.

2. The Nutrient

a) *Selection of Nutrient*

Selection of the nutrient is one of the important factors for successful vascular tissue cultures. The needs of cells vary with their origin by species. Young and old cells of varying type have different requirements.

To obtain monolayers of cells, a substance is added to the liquid nutrient to promote formation of a clot to assure the adhesion of the explant to the support. A single reference has been made to the use of a solid medium. LAZZARINI [1961b] used agar film for the cloning of human and canine aortic cells.

α) Biologic Nutrients

In the living body, the intima is always exposed to the blood stream. Thus, the ideal nutrient for *in vitro* culture would be flowing blood or blood plasma. It would have to be constantly reconstituted. Such arrangement has been used for perfusion studies of arteries. It is not suited to cell cultures. Many investigators have tried a compromise using plasma, serum, or serum ultrafiltrate as the base of a nutrient.

Autologous plasma has been used by CARREL and BURROWS [1910] for cat and dog aortae. BLOOM [1929] cultured guinea pig aortic fibroblasts in heparinized plasma mixed with 9 parts of Tyrode solution and 1 part of guinea pig embryo extract. SHIBUYA [1931] obtained 25% positive cultures from rabbit aortae in Ringer's solution with adrenal extract. SIMMS [1936] and SIMMS and STILLMAN [1937c, 1937d, 1937e] used 1 part of serum and 2 parts of serum UF for studies of lipoid transport by chicken aorta fibroblasts. PARSHLEY *et al.* [1950] used homologous serum or plasma, with Simms' X6 solution or with normal serum UF, for dog aortic cultures. For aortic cell cultures from several species, PARSHLEY *et al.* [1953] added to 1 part of chicken plasma 2 parts of Simms' X6 or Z2 solution or Hanks' solution, or serum UF. INGENITO *et al.* [1958] and RUTSTEIN *et al.* [1958, 1964] grew human aortic fibroblasts in equal parts of chicken plasma and of a mixture of 40% human serum, 20% chick embryo extract, and 40% Hanks' solution. BRANWOOD [1961a] used, as a nutrient for human aortic intima, 2 parts of human serum, 1 part of chick EE, and 2 parts of Hanks' solution. AYKAN [1964] obtained only 1 positive culture from 27 rat aortic explants in a medium consisting of 4 parts of cord serum, 1 part of chick EE, and 1 part of Gey's solution. Results with vascular tissue cultures in biologic nutrients have not been opulent.

β) Chemical Nutrients

Some investigators seek a nutrient which would mimic *in vitro* the *in vivo* environment of intimal cells; others desire a chemically defined medium without a biologic base. Theoretically, cells in a synthetic medium should be ideally suited for metabolic studies. WAYMOUTH [1965] listed 51 chemical nutrients, some of which were designed for a specific cell strain while others were proposed for general use.

Four synthetic nutrients have been used most often for vascular cell cultures: Medium 199 of MORGAN *et al.* [1950], medium NCTC 109 of EVANS *et al.* [1956], medium MB 752/1 of WAYMOUTH [1959], and medium N-16 of PUCK *et al.* [1958] which contains 4% of NCTC 109.

Medium 199 has been used by LAZZARINI [1961d] for human and canine aortic cells—after the addition of 1% peptone and 10% arginine, and by CURTIS and GALVIN [1963]—after the addition of 15 parts of human serum or horse serum, and 7 parts of chick EE. SMITH *et al.* [1965] failed to culture pigeon aortic cells in medium 199, even after addition of 10% calf serum, or 1% peptone and 3 mg% arginine. Pigeon aortic cells grew equally well in NCTC-109—after addition of 10% to 20% horse, calf, bovine or pigeon serum—as in other media. The authors also tried lactoalbumin hydrolysate 0.5% in Hanks' solution, with 10% or 20% bovine serum; chick EE_{50} 2% in Hanks' solution with 10% to 40% pigeon serum; homologous pigeon EE_{50}, 2% to 20% in Hanks' solution with 40% pigeon serum; further, medium BM-752/1 enriched with 10% calf serum.

Medium MB-752/1 was compared with the Eagle's basal medium enriched with 15% of several types of serum by KOKUBU and POLLAK [1960, 1961a]. The growth of aortic fibroblasts in the chemical medium—without additive—was disappointing. LAZZARINI [1962b] enriched synthetic medium with 10% homologous serum and used this 'semi-synthetic' nutrient for the study of lipoprotein transport by human intimal cells.

The N-16 medium was used after addition of 10% fetal calf serum by MORRISON *et al.* [1963] and by MURATA *et al.* [1965] for cultures of chicken aortae. MURATA [1968] used it also for endothelial cells and fibroblasts from Rhesus aortae. LAZZARINI [1962a, 1962d] also employed No. 6 Spinner medium supplemented with inorganic chemicals and, later, HMA-4 medium.

γ) Basal and Essential Nutrients

In spite of the inclusion of purine and pyrimidine compounds, of nucleotides and coenzymes, synthetic media have not proven suitable for vascular cell cultures. The necessity of adding biologicals, such as serum, plasma, or egg extract, defeats the purpose for which the chemically defined media were developed. Two media—the basal medium of EAGLE (BME) [1955], which incorporates Hanks' solution, and the minimum essential medium of EAGLE (MEM) [1959], which incorporates Earle's solution, have been proven superior to other nutrients. Before use, the stock solutions are enriched with

L-glutamine and supplemented with blood serum. Usually, chick embryo extract (EE_{50}) is also added.

The MEM medium, supplemented with 10% fetal calf serum, has been used by MORRISON *et al.* [1963] and by MURATA *et al.* [1965] for culture of chicken aortae in studies of the effects of mucopolysaccharides and lipoids.

The BME medium has been used for rabbit aortic cultures by POLLAK *et al.* [1960 and on], since KOKUBU and POLLAK [1960, 1961] compared it with Waymouth's nutrient. To 70 ml of the stock BME, 15 ml of chick EE_{50}, 15 ml of blood serum, and 0.0146 mg of L-glutamine were added. For rabbit aortae, horse serum was used until 1963; since then, calf serum has been used. For human arteries, human serum was added to the stock solution. Empirically, the chick EE was omitted for culture of smooth muscle cells and the amount of L-glutamine doubled by KASAI and POLLAK [1964a]. At pH 7.2 to 7.6, 90% to 100% positive cultures were obtained from ascending aortae of rabbits. From normal human arteries, POLLAK and ADACHI [1968] obtained up to 60% of endothelial cell cultures and 90% of fibroblast cultures using the BME nutrient. SMITH *et al.* [1965] found the BME nutrient with 10% to 50% calf serum, or with 15% horse serum, and with 15% chick EE_{50} and 0.145 mg of L-glutamine per liter best among the nutrients for the proliferation of pigeon aortic fibroblasts and for the maintenance of these cells for 18 passages. CHOI *et al.* [1968] used BME medium with 10% calf or swine serum for 15 passages of minipig aortic cells.

b) Optimal Nutrients

α) Electrolytes

The balanced salt solution of EARLE is part of the MEM nutrient. The solutions of GEY and GEY [1936], the X6, X7 and Z2 solutions of SIMMS and SANDERS [1942], solutions of EARLE *et al.* [1943] and of HANKS and WALLACE [1949] have been used extensively in vascular tissue culture work.

The transport of electrolytes across the cell membrane plays a role in cell metabolism. Calcium, potassium, sodium, and magnesium ions are located on the uppermost surface and on the innermost layer of the cell membrane, together with protein and mucopolysaccharide molecules, and externally to lipoid and phospholipoid molecules. POLLAK [1968a] suggested that the transmembrane movement of electrolytes may regulate cellular lipoid metabolism. Until pertinent studies of this question have been made, it will be difficult to discuss the choice of electrolyte solutions for vascular tissue cultures. SIMMS and SANDERS [1942] stated that Simms' X6 salt solution has a greater buffering capacity than other balanced salt solutions for arterial fibroblasts and endothelial cells. Magnesium may enhance the growth and adhesiveness of fibroblasts.

β) Hydrogen Ion Concentration

The maintenance of a constant optimal reaction of the nutrient is very important. Universally, Phenol Red is used as an indicator of pH. The reaction of the stock medium without additives, and of the final nutrient after the addition of serum and tissue extracts, is adjusted with 1.4% sodium bicarbonate solution. A pH of 7.6 has been postulated by SIMMS and STILLMAN [1937c, 1937d, 1937e] for chicken aortic fibroblasts. PARSHLEY *et al.* [1950] adjusted the pH from 7.2 to 7.8 for dog aortic cells. Cells from 7 species were grown at pH 7.4 by PARSHLEY and DETERLING [1953]. INGENITO *et al.* [1958] grew human aortic fibroblasts at pH 7.6. LAZZARINI [1959] and KOKUBU and POLLAK [1961a] established a pH of 7.2 to 7.4 as optimal for all their vascular tissue culture work.

γ) Renewal of the Nutrient

To maintain a stable reaction, the nutrient has to be periodically renewed. Usually, this is done as soon as the color of the indicator begins to change from red to yellow. This indicates acidity. Increasing acidity of the nutrient promotes degeneration of cells, according to SIMMS *et al.* [1947]. BLOOM [1929] changed his medium for guinea pig aortae every 6 to 7 days. He washed the cells in Tyrode solution and used 9 parts of Tyrode solution and 1 part of guinea pig embryo extract. He omitted the 3rd component of the nutrient, namely heparinized plasma. This was not a reconstitution of the nutrient, but rather a transplantation of cells. SIMMS [1937] used serum for his primary cultures, serum UF for secondary cultures. PARSHLEY *et al.* [1953] and KOKUBU and POLLAK [1961a] renewed their nutrient twice a week; LAZZARINI [1959] changed it every 4th day, increasing at the time of change the amount of added homologous serum from 10% to 40% and omitting chicken plasma from the original nutrient mixture. BRANWOOD [1961a] replaced the medium after 1, 3, and 7 days, or before the 7th day if the pH had changed earlier. WEXLER and THOMAS [1967] changed the medium every 3 days, and the gas phase every day.

δ) Amino Acids

Amino acids are the most important components of culture media. Cells from different species have different needs. Amino acid requirements vary with the cell type. Because of constant turnover during propagation, the requirements for amino acids also vary with the age of each cell type. Conditions for pure cell lines and for mixed populations in which cells compete for nutrients are not the same. Our knowledge of the variables, however, is superficial.

Various formulae of media vary quantitatively and qualitatively. The BME and MEM media each contain only one-half as many amino acids as the NCTC-109 medium, two-thirds the amount in nutrients 199 and BM 572/1, and three-fourths as many as in N-16 medium.

Commonly, 0.146 mg/l of L-glutamine is added to the BME or MEM media. Although arginine is present in nutrients, LAZZARINI [1961a] added 10% arginine and 1% peptone to medium 199. He referred to this preparation at the 'final' medium for human and canine aortic cells. SMITH *et al.* [1965] used the same formula—i.e. medium 199 with arginine and peptone—for pigeon aortae, with inferior results. This may be an example of the species-dependent requirements of aortic cells.

KOKUBU and POLLAK [1960, 1961a] obtained similar culture results of aortic fibroblasts of rabbits with 15% horse serum supplement and with 12.5% gelatine in physiologic saline. They noted that the 2 additives contained an equal amount of glycine, which fibroblasts apparently require. POLLAK *et al.* [1960] and ENGEL and POLLAK [1961] reported a decrease in the amounts of glycine and valine in the nutrient after 1 week—when fibroblasts dominated the aortic cell population. ENGEL [1961] suggested that, in the case of a nutrient lacking glycine, the cells obtained glycine and also glutamic acid either from the serum additive, from the degradation of serum or EE_{50}, or from synthesis of amino acids. Glucose may be a source of glycine; glutamine may be a source of glutamic acid.

Discussing papers presented by KOKUBU [1961] and by ENGEL [1961], WERTHESSEN [1961] pointed out that glutamine is an essential energy donor for mucopolysaccharide synthesis. SIMMS [1961], discussing the same papers, stated that only 2 amino acids—aspartic acid and glutamine—stimulate the growth of aortic cells, whereas other amino acids are either nonessential or inhibitive to cell growth. In this connection, it is pointed out that the best nutrients for vascular cell cultures—BME and MEM—do not contain aspartic acid. Apparently, the addition of fresh glutamine is sufficient for the manifold functions of this amino acid as a carbon source for other acids and as a limiting factor in MPS synthesis.

ε) Other Components

Multiple substances with the purine ring or pyridine ring—nucleotides, adenylic cycle members, coenzymes, and growth factors—have been incorporated into the synthetic media 199 and NCTC-109. There is no proof that one or more of these substances promote, in any fashion, vascular tissue cultures. Some of the compounds may be harmful: DPN participates in lipogenesis, and Tween 80 is a source of fatty acids. There is contradiction in preparing a complex, protein-free chemically defined nutrient such as NCTC 109, and then recommending the addition of whole egg extract.

η) Vitamins

The whole range of vitamins has been incorporated into the stock media. EAGLE [1955, 1959] included 8 vitamins in his BME and MEM nutrients, with only minor differences between the two. PUCK *et al.* [1958] used 9 vitamins, while WAYMOUTH [1959] used 11. Medium 199 contains 15 vitamins and medium 109 has 17. The addition of vitamins to the mixture of electrolytes and amino acids seems essential. Yet, it can be overdone. The nutrients with fewer vitamins render better results for vascular tissue cultures than those with large numbers. It should be kept in mind that all the mentioned nutrients were devised for nonvascular cells. The vitamins which participate in enzymatic processes—nicotinamide, pantothenate, and riboflavin—are present in all commercially available stock solutions. Research possibilities in the field of vitamins and trace elements as components of nutrients for vascular cells have not been exhausted.

c) Additives

α) Plasma, Serum, Serum Ultrafiltrate

Before chemically defined solutions became available, it was common practice to mix blood fluids with Tyrode solution, Ringer's solution, Gey's solution, or Simms' salt solutions. Even after stock mixtures of amino acids, electrolytes, and vitamins have become popular, some investigators continued to use blood or plasma for vascular cultures.

As it became clear that vascular cells thrive in media to which serum or plasma has been added, it became important to weigh the merits of autologous, homologous, and heterologous plasma, serum or serum UF. The most probing study was made by PARSHLEY *et al.* [1953]. Autologous serum had been expected to be superior to other serum: It was, thrice, but it failed twice with human aortic cells. Autologous serum, in 16.5% and in 25% concentration, was well-suited for the aortic cells of cats and goats, but not for canine cells. Homologous serum was not always better than heterologous serum or plasma. Human placental plasma gave very good results for dog aortic cells. Chicken plasma was inferior to homologous serum for canine

ditives to nutrients. Adrenal extract reduced the dormancy phase for cellular outgrowth from canine aortic explants, but it also promoted fat deposits in the cells. Dog heart extract reduced the lag phase for canine and human cells by from 4% to 10%. In combination with 25% placental serum, 8% dog heart extract increased the number of positive cultures from canine aortae. In combination with 33% dog serum, 5% dog splenic extract increased the number of successful cultures from dog aortae. Cat and monkey aortae were only slightly stimulated by splenic extract; the growth rate of rabbit aortic cells was not promoted at all. Dog splenic extract inhibited goat aortic cells. The dormancy of dog and human cells was shortened by 2 to 7 days, and the growth of fibroblasts was enhanced, by chick embryo extract. SMITH *et al.* [1965] also compared several extracts. They found no differences between the application of 10% to 40% heterologous chick EE and 2% to 20% homologous pigeon EE for the growth and maintenance of pigeon aortic cells.

Chick embryo extract, EE_{50}, was used by INGENITO *et al.* [1958], and by RUTSTEIN *et al.* [1958] for human aortae, by LAZZARINI [1959 and on] for human, chicken, dog, mouse, and rabbit arteries, by KOKUBU and POLLAK [1960 and on] for rabbit and human arteries, by BRANWOOD [1963] for human, and by AYKAN [1964] for rat aortae. SIMMS [1936 and on] has often pointed out that chick embryo extract is not a normal environment for adult cells *in vitro*.

γ) Enzymes

Proteolytic digestion of tissues before transfer to a nutrient was introduced by SIMMS [1936]. He found trypsin and papain growth-stimulating for chicken aortic fibroblasts. SIMMS and STILLMAN [1937c] ascribed this effect to proteolytic digestion of an inhibiting factor of the arterial tissue. They incubated chicken aortae in 0.1% trypsin solution at 20°C/18 hours, and then kept one part of the fluid at 58°C/20 minutes and another part at 100°C/5 minutes. The growth-inhibiting factor was heat-sensitive. They also incubated 15 g of dog and sheep aortae with 20 ml of a 0.2% trypsin solution before testing the fluid on cultures. In contrast to the beneficial effects of trypsin and papain on tissues, lactenin—a bacterial inhibitor in milk—caused a reduction of cell growth. MORRISON *et al.* [1963] kept chicken aortic intima in 1% trypsin at 20°C/14 hours to facilitate separation of cells from the wall. Trypsinized chicken aortic cells were used as 10^6/ml of MEM nutrient by MURATA *et al.* [1966]. In another study, cells were used in 1:300 v/v proportion to nutrient, by MURATA *et al.* [1967].

δ) Antibiotics

All *in vitro* tissue cultures are sensitive to bacterial and viral contamination. BEHBEHANI *et al.* [1965] made the viral susceptibility of aortic cells—derived from 60 biopsies of human atheroma—a theme of a study. The tissue was washed thrice in BME nutrient, minced, cut into 1 to 2 mm pieces, transferred to 3 ml BME with 20% fetal bovine serum per flask and incubated for 7 days at 37°C. After trypsinization, the cells were transplanted to BME media with 20% calf serum. Thirty-two strains grew for 2 generations (F^2), 11 grew to F^6, and 4 grew to F^{30} within 6 months. After 32 to 35 passages, mitosis ceased and the cells degenerated. The cells, which were described as flattened, endothelial polygonal cells by the authors, seem to the critical observer to be typical of old fibroblasts. All the strains proved remarkably susceptible to 30 types of viral agents—especially to rhinovirus. Severe cytopathic changes developed.

Total sterility is a necessity from the moment tissues are removed from the subject until the culture is discarded. It has become routine to add antibiotics to the final nutrient. BRANWOOD [1963] added 1,000 units of penicillin G/ml of nutrient. Others have used penicillin G and dehydrostreptomycin: LAZZARINI [1959 and on] used 50 units of penicillin and 50 μg/ml of streptomycin; INGENITO *et al.* [1958], RUTSTEIN *et al.* [1958], and KOKUBU and POLLAK [1960 and on] used 100 units/ml of penicillin and 50 μg/ml of streptomycin; and WEXLER and THOMAS [1967] applied 5,000 units of each. SIMMS *et al.* [1937 and on] used no antibiotics.

d) Plasma Clot

For stationary cell cultures, an adhesive must be applied to assure the fixation of the explant to the support. Universally, fresh chicken plasma is used as clotting medium. Depending on the size of the explant and on the supporting area to be covered, 2 to 5 drops of plasma are spread over the glass surface onto which the explant is to be placed. PARSHLEY *et al.* [1953] noted that a clot will form between 30 minutes and 2 hours. Generally, flasks, dishes, or test tubes are kept overnight in such a position that the explant lies on the 'floor'. In the morning, they are gently turned so that the 'floor' with the tissue becomes the 'ceiling'. Periodically, as the cultures are examined, the flasks and tubes are inverted or gently rotated to moisten the explant. The plasma clot is removed with the explant.

Vascular cells may adhere better to glassware washed in water which has a high calcium content, according to FREEMAN and MORRISON [1961]. SMITH *et al.* [1965] did not have to use a plasma clot when employing plastic flasks in lieu of glass flasks. The advantage of better adhesion by cells to plastics is outweighed by the difficulty incurred in separating the cells from the support when desired. In the 'sandwich' or 'envelope' preparation of LAZZARINI [1967], the explant was placed between 2 boronsilicate cover slips without adhesive.

Certainly, the use of chicken plasma introduces a 'contaminating' biologic agent. Experiments with gelatine or with resins as adhesives have not been successful. The composition of plasma or other biologic additives, such as tissue extracts and serum, varies from one lot to the next, no matter how large the pool. The effect on tissue metabolism *in vitro*, by serum with different lipoid contents, has been amply demonstrated. Strenuous efforts to eliminate the use of the plasma clot may not be warranted, as long as other biologicals are being added to the basic nutrient.

It may be well to mention that WADA and POLLAK [1967b] and POLLAK and WADA [1966, 1968c] maintained rabbit aortic cells upon transfer from *in vitro* to *in vivo* conditions, using diffusion chambers implanted in rabbits. In the experiments, the aortic cells received no nourishment other than blood plasma diluted by interstitial fluid. It may be desirable to renew efforts of maintaining vascular cells *in vitro* in a biologic environment rather than in synthetic nutrients.

3. Culture Methods

a) Glassware

The choice and handling of explants and the selection of a nutrient—be it of chemical, biologic, or a combined type—are more important than the choice of glassware. However, the results of vascular tissue cultures are influenced by the choice of glassware.

BLOOM [1929], SIMMS [1936 and on], PARSHLEY *et al.* [1950 and on], PARSHLEY and DETERLING [1955], POLLAK *et al.* [1960 and on] used Carrel flasks, mostly the D-30 type. KOKUBU [1961] found miniature Carrel flasks—2.9 cm outside diameter, 0.9 cm outside height, 2.2 mm long neck, 0.8 cm diameter—economical to use and easy to study under the microscope. INGENITO *et al.* [1958], RUTSTEIN *et al.* [1958 and on], and KOKUBU and POLLAK [1961b and on] used Earle's T-15 and T-60 flasks. KOKUBU [1961] noted that prescription bottles are too thick-walled for study, that the walls are not flat, and that the glass was toxic for aortic cells. Nevertheless, such bottles were used by WEXLER and THOMAS [1967]. CURTIS and GALVIN [1963] used 14 ml flasks with 2 ml nutrient; MORRISON *et al.* [1963 and on] used 30 ml flasks with 5 ml media and 1- to 2-liter bottles. SMITH *et al.* [1965] worked with 3-oz bottles and Earle's T-15 flasks. Milk dilution bottles with 10 ml of cell suspension and Leighton tubes with 1.5 ml cell suspension were used by CHOI *et al.* [1968]. Leighton tubes were also used by MORRISON *et al.* [1963], and by POLLAK and ADACHI [1968]. ROBERTSON [1967a] equipped Leighton tubes with perforated screw caps and with biologically inert siliastic diaphragms for gas phase studies.

SMITH *et al.* [1965] preferred Falcon plastic flasks of the T-15 type to glass flasks. POLLAK *et al.* [1960] found disadvantages in the Falcon flasks. On dismembering, the surface supporting the cells can be used for examination as a slide; however, it can be used for only a single staining. Cells have been grown on dacron sheets by FABRIZIO [1961]. Cellophane and filter paper have been used as supports in nonvascular tissue culture work.

Many investigators have experimented with various glass and plastic Petri dishes. POLLAK *et al.* [1962b] used hanging drop slides, placed on a heated stage, to monitor mitosis and phagocytosis by periodic observation and cinemicrophotography. Perfusion chambers were used in similar manner to study the effects of nicotine and cigarette smoke condensate by POLLAK [1961 and on]. This technique, like most of the procedures in vascular tissue culture work, has been demonstrated by ADACHI and his technical assistants in a motion picture by POLLAK and BURNS [1965].

b) Temperature, Humidity, Gas Phase

Mammalian cells grow best at body temperature. *In vitro*, the cells are sensitive to temperature fluctuations. The incubator has to be kept between 37.5°C and 38°C, and the doors have to be opened and closed swiftly. POLLAK [1963] noted that following an electric power failure of 6½ hours, and a temperature drop to 20°C, the growth of all vascular cells in flasks and tubes had ceased.

Vascular cells are also sensitive to light and to dryness. The humidity within an incubator is usually constant and does not need regulation. Drying of the explant and cells can be avoided by turning the flasks and tubes daily. For this reason, Petri dishes are not suitable for tissue cultures. Rotating drums for roller tubes, and flat-surfaced rotators for slides and flasks, will keep cells sufficiently moist. The speed of such devices must be regulated, since excessive motion can disrupt cell coats and cells.

A constant stream of cooled air compensates for the excessive heat generated by the bulbs used in time-lapse cinemicrophotography, according to BURNS [1964]. If vascular cells *in vitro* are sensitive to light, it was not observed during a 5-day time-lapse cinemicrophotography.

The importance of maintaining a proper gas phase has often been stressed. However, few reports include information about the gas phase. SIMMS *et al.* [1937 and on] used 2 to 4% CO_2 in air at all times to prevent inactivation of the 'A' factor. KOKUBU and POLLAK [1961b] and KOIDE *et al.* [1963] compared air with a mixture of 95% O_2 and 5% CO_2 but found no differences in the culture results. Cells are exposed to air during inoculation or during renewal of the nutrient. An artificial gas phase can reach the cells in tubes or flasks or slides only if stoppers or seals have been perforated by injection needles. ROBERTSON [1967a] used perforated screw caps with diaphragms to permit access of the gas to the cells in Leighten tubes for his studies of the influence of oxygen tension on aortic cells. WEXLER and THOMAS [1967] renewed the gas phase—95% air and 5% CO_2—daily for their work with rat aortic fibroblasts.

4. Methods of Observation

a) Morphologic Methods

α) Unstained Preparations

Hanging-drop slides, flasks, and test tubes are examined under the microscope to ascertain earliest outgrowth of cells from the explant, to follow the spreading of the cells, to identify cells in a mixed population, and to plot growth curves. Simple light microscopy is used, under various magnifications. Phase and phase-contrast microscopy, continous, time-lapse, and stop-motion cinephotomicrography are used to study and record mitosis, phagocytosis, and the effect of additives in cytopharmacologic and cytotoxicologic experiments.

BURNS [1964] established some criteria for cinephotomicrography. To obtain a smooth picture of phagocytosis, frames have to be taken at 2-second intervals; for mitosis, a 10-second interval will suffice. To record the primary outgrowth of cells from an aortic explant, 90-second intervals are used. The electron microscope has been employed by LAZZARINI [1959 and on] for study of the microvilli at the cell membrane of aortic cells, and by CHOI *et al.* [1968] to record the minimal changes in minipig aortic cells induced by hypercholesteremic swine serum. Fluorescent antimonkey actomysin globulin has been used by KAO *et al.* [1968] to identify Rhesus aortic smooth muscle cells. Electrophoresis of cultured cells has not been utilized.

β) Stained Slides

Vital and supravital staining of vascular cells was done by SHIBUYA [1931] with carmine, and by KOIDE and POLLAK [1963a] with Neutral Red and with Janus Green. Bouin's, Helly's, Müller's, and Zenker's fluid, buffered formalin solution, and osmium tetraoxide have been used as fixatives for vascular cells.

Many different stains have been applied to slides prepared from vascular cell cultures. The May-Grünwald-Giemsa stain has become most popular to visualize cytoplasmic and nuclear details. Pollak's trichrome stain proved suitable for the demonstration of myofilaments in smooth muscle cells.

For the study of lipoids, Nile blue sulfate, Sudan III, Sudan IV–Oil Red O, Sudan Black B, and the Lieberman-Burchard reaction in the Schultz modification have been used. Slides have been stained with osmium and have been studied under polarized light. A variety of special stains has been employed to demonstrate cytochemically various enzymes. In all such work, photomicrography has been used to secure permanent records.

b) Physiologic Methods

In contrast to morphologic methods, procedures may be applied which can be called physiologic methods. They can be applied to nutrient as well as to cells.

Autoradiography has been used to follow the incorporation of radioactive materials into cells. LAZZARINI [1963a] used this method to study the uptake of S^{35}, MURATA *et al.* [1965, 1966] to study uptake of ^{3}H-thymidine and ^{3}H-uridine, MURATA *et al.* [1967] for Na-acetate-C^{14}, MURATA [1968] for ^{14}C-cholesterol, ROBERTSON [1967a] for labeled cholesterol and phospholipoids, and CHOI *et al.* [1968] to study ^{14}C-glycine and ^{3}H-thymidine uptake.

More often, utilization of radioactive chemicals has been studied by liquid scintillation spectrophotometry of the nutrient and of tissue extracts. This has been applied to the study of lipoids and of mucopolysaccharides. Microsomal fractions of aortic cells, after gradient ultracentrifugation of cell suspensions, were analyzed by LAZZARINI [1962c, 1963a, 1963b].

Most investigators have used cultures with mixed cell populations, but few have paid attention to the composition of the populations, to changes occurring with the aging of cultures and of individual cell types—in summary, to factors which influence the results of investigations.

MURATA *et al.* [1967b] pointed out that different generations of the same culture differed with regard to the incorporation of labeled uridine and thymidine; in addition, they had different growth rates. CHOI *et al.* [1968] reported that the sensitivity of cells to hypercholesteremic serum decreased with subsequent generations of cells. These facts must be considered when interpreting comparative results.

D. Quantitative Aspects of Cell Cultures

Variations caused by the choice of explants, nutrients, and other culture conditions influence the quantitative features of vascular tissue cultures, such as the number of successful cultures or the number of colonies, as well as the qualitative aspects, such as the make-up of cell populations.

1. Success of Cultures

Information about the number of successful vascular tissue cultures is not plentiful. BLOOM [1929] referred to the outgrowth of 'a few cells' from guinea pig aortae. DETERLING and PARSHLEY [1953] obtained 4 positive cultures from 6 canine aortic explants removed within 1 hour after death. Using fresh dog aortae, PARSHLEY and DETERLING [1953] obtained 96% positive cultures with many fibroblasts and a few endothelial cells. PARSHLEY *et al.* [1953] used 188 segments of fresh aortae of 6 rabbits, 4 cats, 1 goat, and 1 monkey. All yielded positive results within 2 to 8 days. However, 16 human aortae yielded only 56% positive cultures. PARSHLEY and DETERLING [1955] obtained 16 positive cultures with 256 colonies from 1388 pieces of 83 explants of fresh canine aortae. Whole-thickness explants gave better results than explants consisting only of intima and inner media. AYKAN [1964] reported 1 good and 3 feeble cultures of fibroblasts from 27 tubes with rat aortic explants. Since heart explants gave comparable results, it seems that the author's limited success may have been due to the methodology, namely to the choice of nutrient.

KOKUBU and POLLAK [1961a] reported on the number of successful cultures of rabbit aortae and myocardial cells. Cardiac cells grew more easily than aortic cells. With BME nutrient as a base, culture results were comparable upon addition of rabbit, horse, or human serum. Chicken serum did not promote cell growth. Growth in nutrient without serum was poor (table II). There was a gradient along the course of the rabbit aortae, similar to that recorded by PARSHLEY *et al.* [1953] for canine aortae.

Table II. Positive cultures from rabbit aortae and heart

Serum	Rabbit		Horse		Human		Chicken		None		Totals	
Ascending	9 of	10	6 of	10	8 of	10	5 of	10	5 of	10	33 of	50
Thoracic	5	9	5	9	3	9	2	9	2	9	17	45
Abdominal	1	9	2	9	1	9	2	9	2	9	8	45
All aorta	15	28	13	28	12	28	9	28	9	28	58	140
Heart	6 of	6	5 of	6	6 of	6	6 of	6	3 of	5	25 of	29

Table III. Positive cultures from two series of rabbit aortae

Days after inoculation	1	2	3	4	5	6	7	8	9	10	11	12	Totals		Cholesterol
Ascending			1	9	11	2					1		24 of	24	normo-
	4	8	7	4									23	24	hyper-
Thoracic				1	3	11	12		1			1	29 of	30	normo-
	1	5	4	5	4	5	2						26	26	hyper-
Abdominal				1	3	2	5	1			6	2	26 of	28	normo-
		1	1	5	7	6	3			1	1		25	25	hyper-
All aorta			1	11	17	15	17	1	1		7	3	73 of	82	normo-
	5	14	12	14	11	11	5			1	1		74	74	hyper-

Table IV. Lag phase of vascular cell types by origin of explants

Cell type	Species	Dormancy Days	References and footnotes
Endothelial	cat	2	HERZOG and SCHOPPER, 1931
		2	PARSHLEY *et al.*, 1953
	chicken	8–12	LAZZARINI, 1959[1]
		8	MORRISON *et al.*, 1963[2]
	dog	8–22	LAZZARINI, 1961 b, 1962 b, 1962 e
		3– 5	PARSHLEY *et al.*, 1950
		4	PARSHLEY and DETERLING, 1953[3]
		2– 3	HERZOG and SCHOPPER, 1931; PARSHLEY *et al.*, 1953
	goat	2	PARSHLEY *et al.*, 1953
	man	28–42	LAZZARINI, 1959
		21–28	INGENITO *et al.*, 1958[4]
		14–21	PARSHLEY *et al.*, 1953[3]

Table IV. (Continuation)

Cell type	Spezies	Dormancy Days	References and footnotes
		8–21	LAZZARINI, 1961b, 1962b, 1962e
		6	POLLAK and ADACHI, 1968
		2– 3	BRANWOOD, 1961a, 1963[5]
	minipig	2– 3	CHOI *et al.*, 1968a, 1968b; FLORENTIN *et al.*, 1968
	monkey	4	PARSHLEY *et al.*, 1953
	mouse	7–21	LAZZARINI, 1959[6]
	rabbit	1– 2	SHIBUYA, 1931; KASAI and POLLAK, 1964
Fibroblasts	cat	3	CARREL and BURROWS, 1910
		2	PARSHLEY *et al.*, 1953
	chicken	8–21	LAZZARINI, 1959[1]
		3– 5	SIMMS, 1936[7]
		1	SIMMS, 1939[1]
	dog	10	DETERLING *et al.*, 1953[8]
		4	PARSHLEY *et al.*, 1953; PARSHLEY and DETERLING, 1953[9]
		3	CARREL and BURROWS, 1910
	goat	2	PARSHLEY *et al.*, 1953
	man	28–42	LAZZARINI, 1959
		21–28	INGENITO *et al.*, 1958
		14–21	PARSHLEY *et al.*, 1953[3]
		8	POLLAK and ADACHI, 1968
		6	BRANWOOD, 1961a, 1963
	monkey	4	PARSHLEY *et al.*, 1953
	mouse	7–21	LAZZARINI, 1959
	rabbit	21–28	LAZZARINI, 1959
		5	KASAI and POLLAK, 1964
		2– 3	SHIBUYA, 1931
		2	POLLAK and ADACHI, 1968
Myocytes	rabbit	12–14	KASAI and POLLAK, 1964a[10,11]
	man	15–17	POLLAK and ADACHI, 1968
Macrophages	rabbit	1– 2	KOKUBU and POLLAK, 1961c; KASAI *et al.*, 1964[12]
	man	9	POLLAK and ADACHI, 1968[12]
Mesenchymal	man	5	BRANWOOD, 1961a, 1963
Heart cells	man	28	INGENITO *et al.*, 1958
	rabbit	2	KOKUBU, 1961; KOKUBU and POLLAK, 1961a

[1] embryo, [2] trypsinized before planting, [3] as long as 14–21 days, [4] only 5% endothelial cells, [5] intima only, [6] lag of endothelial cells shorter than of fibroblasts, [7] 1 year old, [8] longer, if first frozen, [9] after 48 hours of refrigeration, [10] uterine, 2–4 days (comparison), [11] atherosclerotic, 15 to 17 days, [12] fat-laden cells.

In another study, KOKUBU and POLLAK [1961b, 1961c] charted, every day for 12 days, the number of positive results for cells grown from 3 aortic sectors. The results for explants from normocholesteremic rabbits reflected the outgrowth of 2 cell types, endothelial cells and fibroblasts. The results for explants from hypercholesteremic rabbits differed because of the early and opulent appearance of a 3rd cell type, a fat-laden cell. The growth gradient along the course of the aortae was accentuated because of the fat-laden cells from the proximal aortae with atherosclerotic plaques (table III).

2. Dormancy

Many reports have been made on the period of dormancy—the lag phase—of vascular cells (table IV).

The lag phase of each cell type depends on the origin by species. For example, all human cells have a longer dormancy than their corresponding rabbit cells. For each type, the lag phase depends upon the distance from the surface of the explant. This accounts for the longer lag phase of fibroblasts in comparison with endothelial cells, and it accounts for the longer lag phase of smooth muscle cells compared with the other two cell types, and also for the longer dormancy of myocytes beneath a thickened atherosclerotic intima-subintima when compared with that of myocytes from the normal artery. Improvement in techniques has led to the reports of shorter periods. For example, the lag for human endothelial cells was reported by LAZZARINI as 28 to 42 days and as 8 to 21 days, in 1959 and 1961, respectively.

3. Growth Values

Few investigators have paid attention to the growth values of vascular cells *in vitro*. Nutritional requirements and metabolic functions fluctuate with the absolute number of cells in a culture at a given moment and with the composition of the population which is never stagnant.

The growth values can be studied in several ways. PARSHLEY and DETERLING [1955] counted cells in a hemocytometer. To date, electronic cell counters have not been used. MORRISON *et al.* [1965] supplemented hemocytometer counts by determining the total cell volume as cytocrit value. They also evaluated cell growth by the dry weight of cells.

The growth values (GV) were originated by SIMMS and STILLMAN [1937c] and were later modified by PARSHLEY and DETERLING [1950]:

$$GV = \frac{\text{Number of cells per flask}}{\text{Number of explants per flask}}$$

KOKUBU and POLLAK [1961a] trypsinized a total cell population and mixed the washed cells, resuspended in physiologic saline, with an equal volume of 0.1% Crystal Violet in 0.1 M citric acid. A scale of 7 values was best suited for the study of aortic cells:

GV 0 no cells
1 1 to 50 new cells
2 51 to 100 new cells
3 101 to 1000 new cells
4 0.1×10^4 to 1×10^4 new cells
5 1×10^4 to 6×10^4 new cells
6 6×10^4 to 10×10^4 new cells
7 more than 10×10^4 new cells

To count the different cell types in a mixed population, KOKUBU and POLLAK [1961c] prepared multiple negatives and enlarged positives of photomicrographs of cultures. Cells were counted by projecting the negatives on a screen, or by circling the cells on prints using multicolored pencils.

4. Growth Curves

By plotting daily growth values, one arrives at the growth curve for both cell population and individual cell types. Such curves yielded information about the lag phase, the speed of proliferation, the maximum growth value, aging and longevity, and synergistic and competitive growth.

In analyzing and comparing growth curves, one must know the type and position of the explant, the proportion between the size of the explant and the amount of nutrient, and the choice and renewal time of the nutrient. Growth curves are influenced by many environmental factors, although to differing extents.

Growth curves for rabbit aortic cells were plotted by KOKUBU [1960] and by KOKUBU and POLLAK [1961b, 1961c] from growth values obtained from explants of normal sectors and explants of sectors with experimental atherosclerotic lesions. The published material has become obsolete when the cell called 'intermediate' was identified as an endothelial cell and the

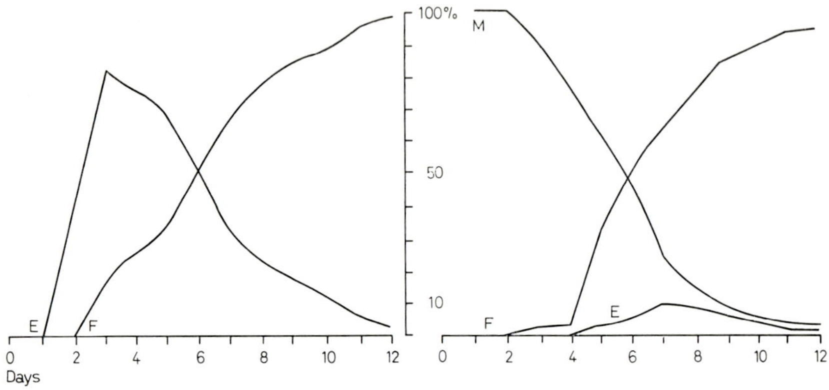

Fig. 1. Growth curves for cells of primary cultures from (left) intact and (right) atherosclerotic rabbit aortae. E = endothelial cells; F = fibrocytes; M = macrophages.

'modified endothelial cell' obtained from plaques was identified as a fat-laden macrophage (fig. 1).

The growth curves for fibroblasts from intact and from atherosclerotic aortae are similar. Endothelial cells from intact aortae proliferated vigorously and maximum growth values were reached shortly; then, the growth curve began to decline and crossed the ascending curve of fibroblasts. In the 12-day-old culture—the explant had been removed 48 hours after planting—fibroblasts dominated the field. The appearance of endothelial cells from atherosclerotic aortae was delayed, their proliferation was slight and brief. The investigators ascribed this to the early appearance of fat-laden cells which, in the plaque, are located above endothelial cells. By the time that the endothelial cells made their first appearance, the number of fibroblasts was large enough to prevent the proliferation of endothelial cells. Fat-laden cells did not reproduce and their number declined from the first day on.

Branwood [1961a] plotted curves for cells grown from pellicle preparations of human aortic intima. His curves were remarkably similar to those prepared by Kokubu [1961] for rabbits' cells.

Growth curves for rabbit aortic cells, for cells from the aortae of human newborns, from medium-sized human arteries, and human adult aortae were drawn by Pollak and Adachi [1968] (fig. 2). The nearly identical curves for rabbit aortae and human infant aortae was ascribed to comparable wall thickness of these vessels. The growth curves for adult human arterial cells were by far not as steep as that for infant aortae. Adult human aortic cells grew poorly.

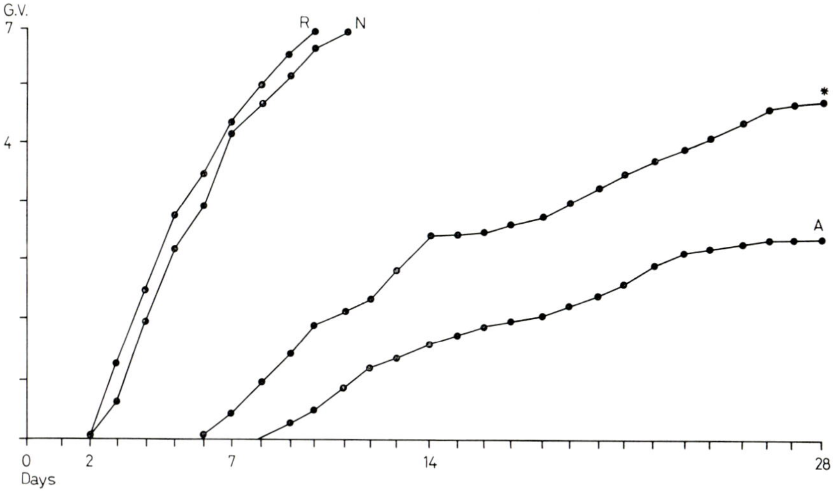

Fig. 2. Growth values (G.V.) and growth curves for cell populations in primary cultures of (R) rabbit aortae, (N) newborn human aortae, (*) popliteal, femoral, and tibial arteries (composite), and (A) adult human aortae. [Figure 9 in POLLAK, O.J. and ADACHI, T., 1968; reproduced with permission of S. Karger, Basel.]

5. Differentiation, Dedifferentiation

The analysis and interpretation of growth curves leads to a discussion of cell metamorphosis. All those who have cultured vascular endothelial cells and fibroblasts have acknowledged the earlier appearance of endothelial cells. All have observed the early disappearance of endothelial cells, and the gradual dominance of fibroblasts in mixed cultures. KOKUBU and POLLAK [1961b, 1961c] ascribed this phenomenon to differences in the lag phase—which they explained by the cellular topography—, the different rates of proliferation, and competitive growth.

Many investigators have misinterpreted the change in cell population as a metamorphosis of endothelial cells into fibroblasts. MAXIMOW [1925] thought that it is not feasible to distinguish the two cell types grown from pia mater. Intracellular bridges were viewed as evidence of metamorphosis of cells. SILBERBERG [1929] called the growth of endothelial cells from pia, choroid plexus, and veins; in actuality, he described fibroblasts. He mistakenly stated that the two cell types resemble each other and that endothelial cells transform into fibroblasts. HERZOG and SCHOPPER [1931] subscribed to the concept of dedifferentiation of endothelial cells into fibroblasts and of fibroblasts into macrophages. SHIBUYA [1931] identified endothelial cells from rabbit aortic explants, but ascribed the change in cell population on the 5th or 6th day to the transformation of endothelial cells into fibroblasts, histiocytes, and multinucleated giant cells. His reference to liquefaction of the nutrient, which he thought typical for endothelial cells, suggests a contamination of his cultures. PEIRCE *et al.* [1949] found the distinction between endothelial cells and fibroblasts too difficult to determine, and he did not pursue this problem.

The identification of cells has become easier with the improvement of methodology. At one point, PARSHLEY *et al.* [1953] suspected a change of endothelial cells into fibroblasts. In his first report of experiments with cells grown from adult human aortae and from chick embryo aortae, LAZZARINI [1955] could not tell endothelial cells from fibroblasts. In subsequent studies, he had no difficulties with this. The categoric statement by LAZZARINI [1959, 1961] that there is no transformation in either direction between the 2 cell types has been supported by KOIDE *et al.* [1963] who monitored rabbit aortic cells by time-lapse cinephotomicrography over a 5-day period.

BRANWOOD [1961a, 1963] devoted much thought to the problem of metamorphosis. In cultures from human aortic intima, triangular-polygonal cells appeared at the periphery in 5-day-old cultures. He labeled such cells as 'transitional', mesenchymal, or primitive reticular. He considered them the result of the 1st phase of dedifferentiation of endothelial cells. The 2nd phase of dedifferentiation, toward a simplified state, was the transformation of transitional cells into fibroblasts. He referred to this phase as 'nomicoplastic fibroplasia' or 'fibroblastic nomicoplasia'. He claimed that this process could be blocked by adding to the nutrient hyperlipemic serum. He further stated that the transformation of endothelial cells resumed when the lipoid-laden cells were washed and transferred to new nutrient. HAUST [1961], discussing such reports, suggested that the term 'dedifferentiation' should not be used and that one should refer to the 'reversal' of a mature

---

Fig. 3. Rabbit aortic cells appearing as 'round' cells during mitosis. Phase contrast; time-lapse cinephotomicrography. *A.* Endothelial cells (×50). Intervals between frames a–f, 4½′, 6′, 3′, 1½′, and 6′. [Reduced from figure 5 in BURNS, D.A., 1964; reproduced with permission of Lea and Febiger, Philadelphia.] *B.* Fibrocytes (×50). Intervals between frames a–h, 4½′, 6′, 1½′, 3′, 6′, 6′, and 6′. [Reduced from figure 8 in KOIDE, R.; POLLAK, O.J. and BURNS, D.A., 1963; reproduced with permission of Elsevier, Amsterdam.]

A

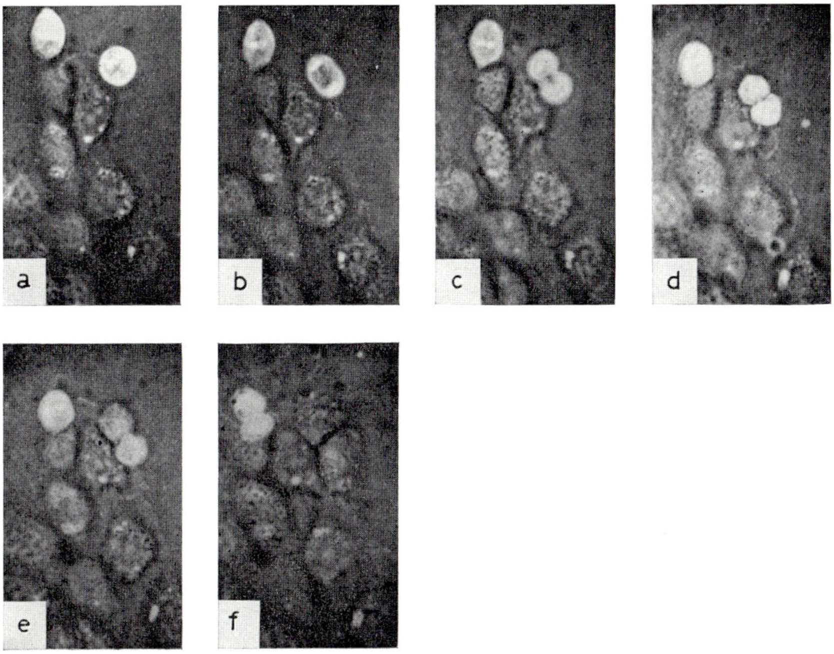

B

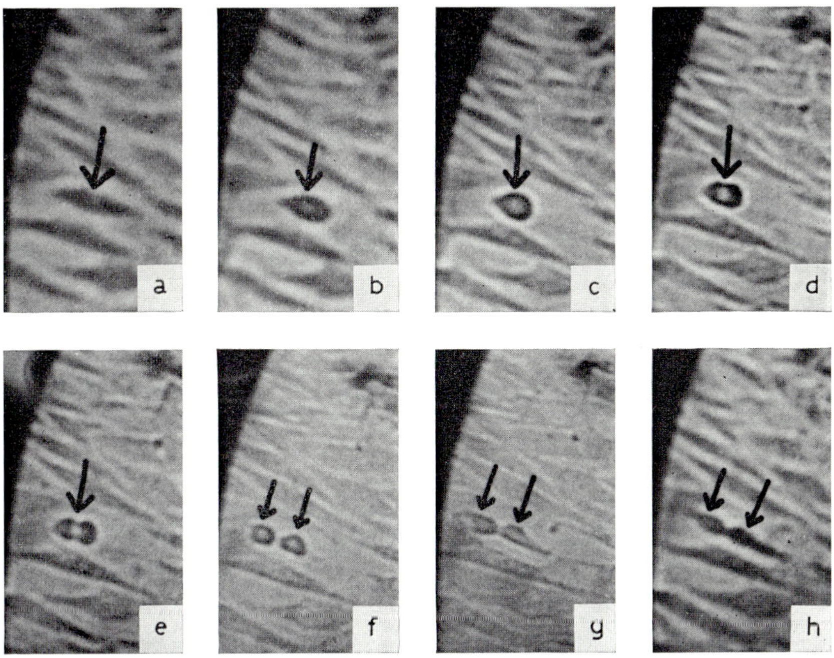

cell to a precursor stage. Dedifferentiation of myocytes of minipig aortic media was suggested by FRITZ *et al.* [1969] but not proven.

Investigators who suggest a transformation of cells speak of a change from 'round' cells to 'spindle-shaped' cells. In contrast, POLLAK *et al.* [1962], KOIDE *et al.* [1963], and KASAI *et al.* [1964] discussed the appearance of 'round forms' in mixed cell cultures. They observed that endothelial cells and fibroblasts become rounded or spheric (a) when exposed to cytotoxins, (b) when loaded with lipoid granules, (c) in the course of degenerative aging, and (d) at the height of mitosis (figs. 3A and B). The fat-laden macrophage is the only truly spheric (round) cell. And this cell is the only cell which results from lipoid loading of cells of varied origin.

6. Nomenclature

The initial difficulties in distinguishing between endothelial cells and fibroblasts were compounded by the overlap of the growth curves of the 2 cell types. The appearance of cells which did not match the morphologic characteristics of either of the 2 types further complicated the task of identifying the cells.

Instead of a definite designation of cells as either endothelial or fibroblastic, LAZZARINI [1959–1963] spoke of 'cytotypes I and II'. The descriptions and illustrations matched those of endothelial cells and fibroblasts, respectively. KOKUBU [1961] and KOKUBU and POLLAK [1961b–1963] referred to spindle cells as type I, to a 'transitional' cell type as II, to polyhedric-round cells as type III, and to lipoid-bearing round cells as type IIIa. Type II was later identified as an aging endothelial cell, type IIIa as the 'foam cell'. The 'transitional' cell was also described by BRANWOOD [1961a]. ROBERTSON [1967] introduced 3 new terms: Intimal cells became 'intimacytes'; endothelial cells with lipoid became 'atherocytes'. Fibrocytes became 'fibrophils'. These terms seem confusing and redundant. It is by no means certain that all fat-laden cells derive from endothelial cells. It may be desirable to reserve the term 'intima' for the endothelial cell layer and the term 'subintima' for the subendothelial layer. In such case, one would have to call the endothelial cells 'intimacytes' and the fibrocytes would become 'subintimacytes'. It is best to forget new terminology and to use the well-defined designations—endothelial cells, fibrocytes, myocytes, and fat-laden macrophages—for the 4 types of cells which can be isolated from blood vessels *in vitro*.

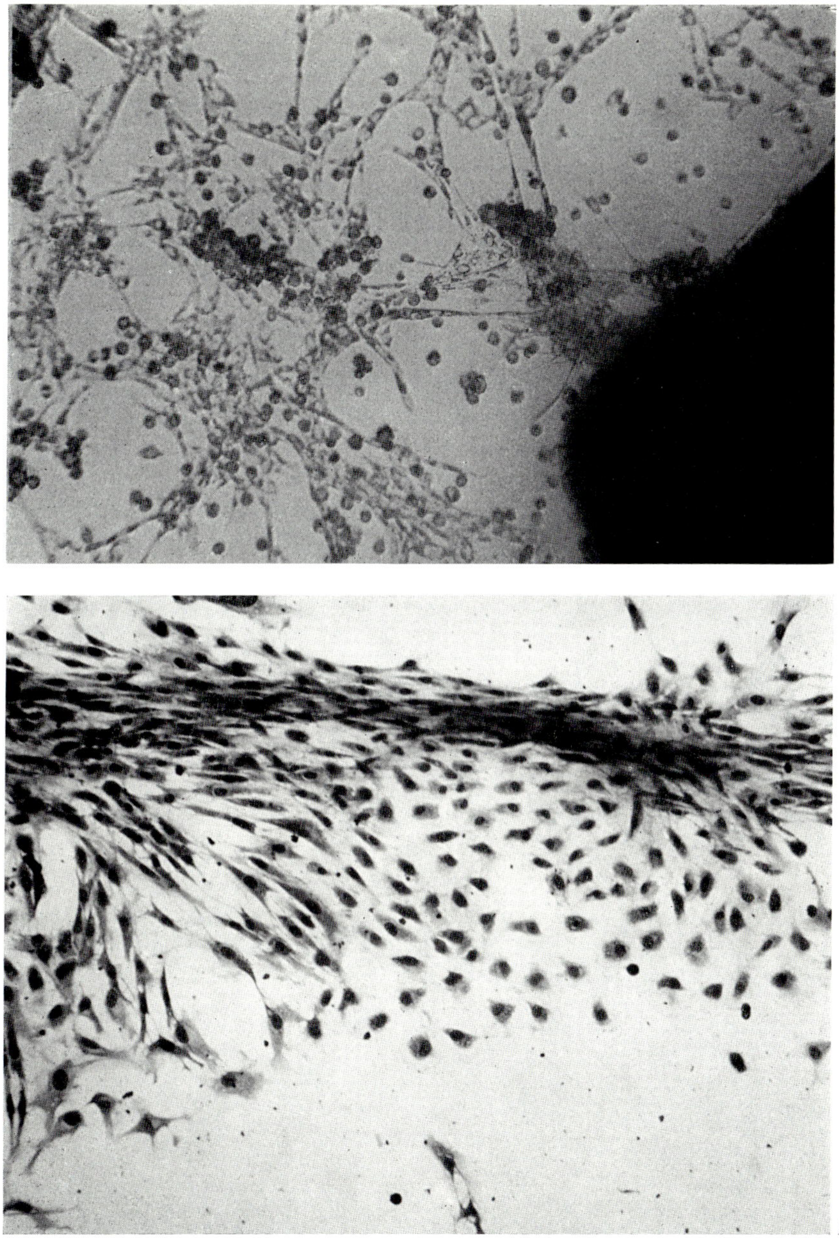

A

B

Fig. 4. A. Position of fat-laden macrophages (small, dark, round) in relation to an explant from rabbit aortic plaque. Culture, 3 days old. Hematoxylin-eosin stain (× 10). *B.* Position of endothelial cells (polyhedric) and fibrocytes (spindle-shaped) in relation to an explant from rabbit aorta. Culture, 5 days old. Hematoxylin-eosin stain (× 11).

7. Cell Kinetics

The changes which occur in mixed cell populations from vascular explants may be called cell kinetics. A stationary cell culture is not a static culture.

Explants are usually positioned near the center of the support. After dormancy, endothelial cells grow in form of buds on the intimal surface of the explant; then, they form mosaics or sheets of fairly uniform size. Slowly, they move away from the explant, in amoeboid fashion. Fibrocytic outgrowth occurs in palm-like cords, as ferns, or as fringed chains. Fibrocytes have a forward movement reminiscent of flagellates; they migrate toward the periphery.

The growth zone around the explant is about 0.5 mm in 1 day, 2 mm in 5 days, and 3 mm in 7 days. Spreading of cells and migration are subject to environmental influences. Cells flatten with aging and upon the addition of hyperlipemic serum or chicken serum to the nutrient. Due to variations in the dormancy, a mixed population develops within 2 to 8 days, depending on the origin of the explant by species and by anatomic site.

The attachement of cells is also influenced by many factors. The cohesiveness-promoting 'D' factor of serum has been studied extensively, by SIMMS and STILLMAN [1937a], and SIMMS *et al.* [1947].

To differing degrees, all cells lose their connection with the explant. Macrophages detach immediately and are seen scattered between other cells (fig. 4A). Endothelial cells detach somewhat later, first from the explant and then from each other. After dissociation, they are seen isolated at some distance from the explant. Fibrocytes often remain connected to the explant, positioned at a 90° angle or as radiating cords at various angles (fig. 4B). Smooth muscle cells also begin to grow at a right angle to the explant (fig. 5A). They do not detach, but spread in syncytial fashion toward the periphery.

Fig. 5. A. Position of smooth muscle cells in relation to an explant from rabbit aorta. Culture, 12 days old. Pollak's trichrome stain (×1000). *B.* Formation of a cell cord by smooth muscle cells from rabbit aorta. Culture, 14 days old. Pollak's trichrome stain (×100). [Figure 6 in KASAI, T. and POLLAK, O.J., 1964a; reproduced with permission of Springer, Berlin/Göttingen/Heidelberg.]

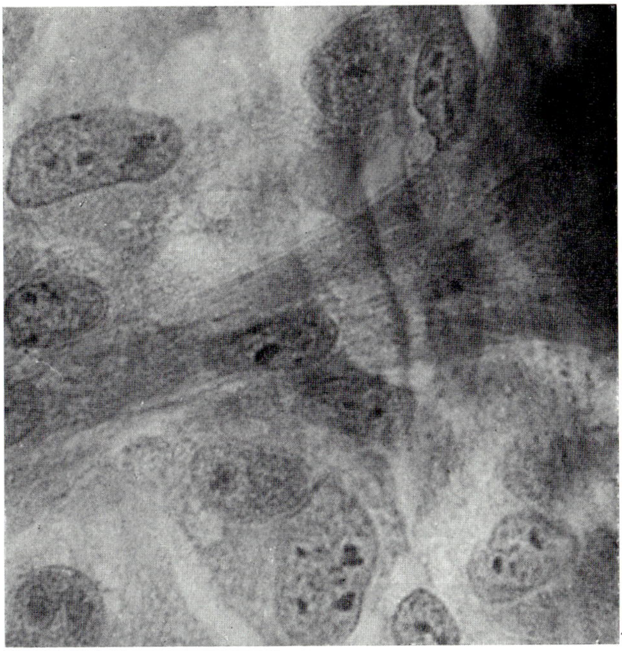

A

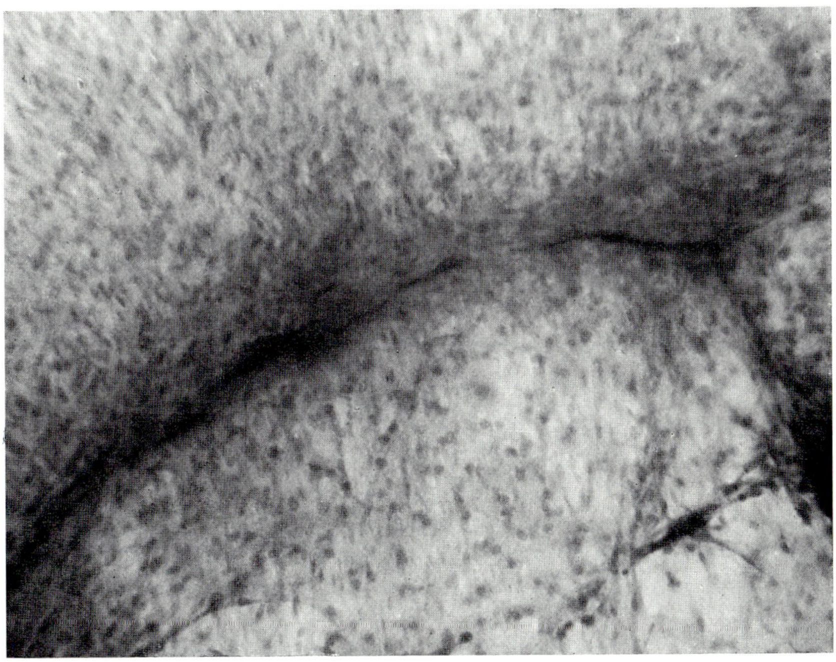

B

Agglutination of vascular cells is caused by a change in osmotic pressure, which, for mammalian cells, optimally equals a 0.8% sodium chloride solution. More often, the grouping of cells, especially of fat-laden cells, is not agglutination in an immunologic sense, but aggregation or agglomeration due to the attraction and interaction of cells of the same type. Clumping of cells of different types is only seen under the influence of toxins. In addition to self-aggregation, clumping can be expedited by physical forces such as centrifugation, rotation, radiation, or by chemicals such as polyvinylalcohol or globulin.

Physiologic manifestations of cell life are somewhat related to cell kinetics. BLOOM [1929] claimed that guinea pig aortic cells formed elastic, reticulum, and collagen fibers in 15- to 17-day-old cultures. HERZOG and SCHOPPER [1931] observed fibrils between the endothelial cells in 5- to 6-day-old cultures. They thought that such fibers were formed by endothelial cells. BRANWOOD mentioned collagen formation by human aortic fibroblasts [1961a] and, at the endstage of fibroblastic nomicoplasia, reticulin formation [1963]. The development of a collagen cap as a bridge across the ring-shaped explant of a rat aorta has been described by WEXLER and THOMAS [1967]. Much the same has been demonstrated by WADA and POLLAK [1967b] for *in vivo* cultures of rabbit aortic explants, in which collagen accumulated beneath the endothelium.

Reaggregation, *in vitro*, of vascular cells into chimærae has not been attempted. Closest to such attempt is the aggregation of smooth muscle cells into a cell cord. KASAI and POLLAK [1964] demonstrated that such smooth muscle cords gave a typical staining reaction for muscle (fig. 5B).

Another tendency toward chimæric organization was observed by KASAI and POLLAK [1964], and by POLLAK and KASAI [1964]. A layer of smooth muscle cells grew beneath a layer of fibroblasts in a rectangular manner (fig. 6). The phenomenon was seen in cultures of aortae and of veins from rabbit and from man. The orientation of the 2 cell types imitates the natural architecture of the vascular wall. The outcome of an experiment in which endothelial cells would be added to the meshwork is currently only a topic of speculation.

Fig. 6. Symbiotic growth of rabbit aortic fibrocytes (in focus in figure 6A) and myocytes (in focus in figure 6B). Culture, 18 days old. Pollak's trichrome stain (×850). [Figures 5A and B in KASAI, T. and POLLAK, O.J., 1964a; reproduced with permission of Springer, Berlin/Göttingen/Heidelberg.]

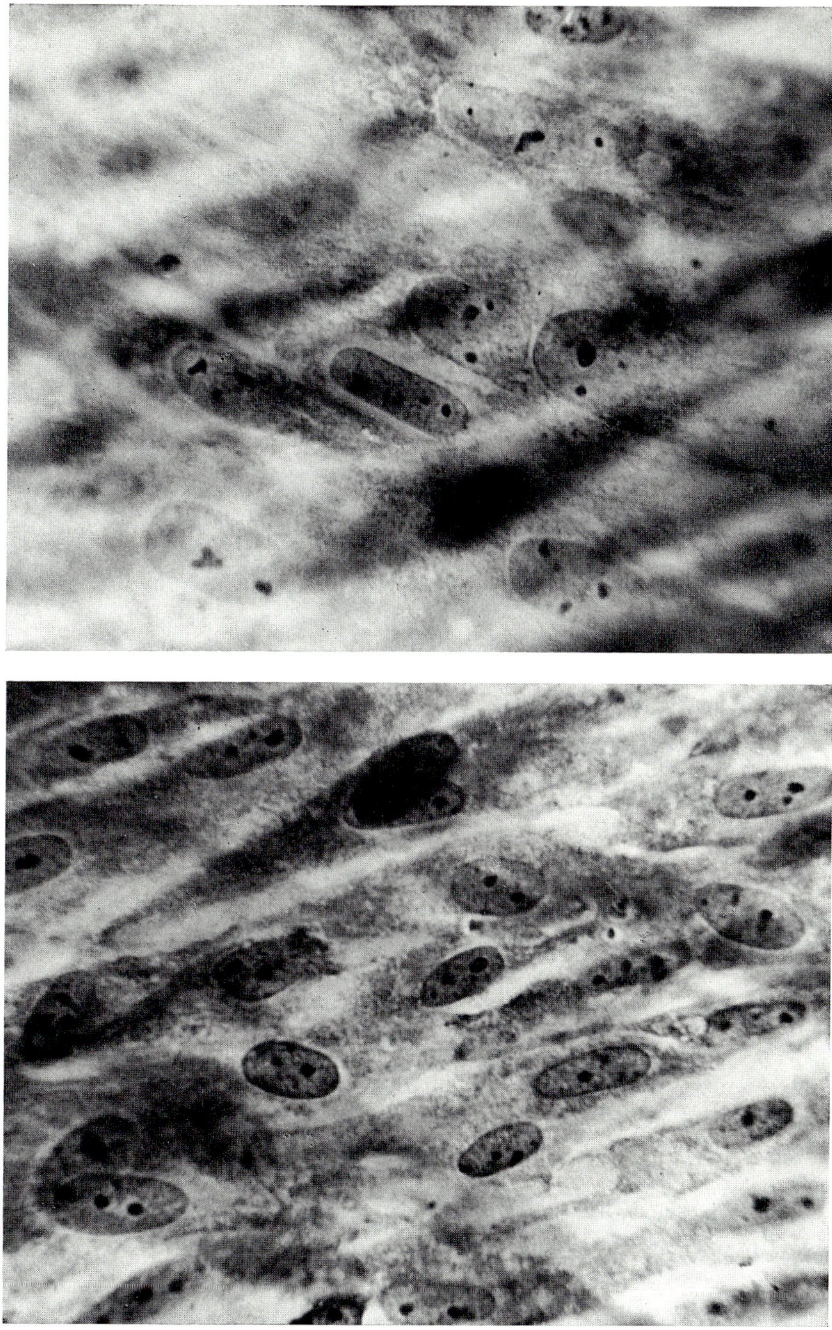

A

B

8. Stimulation of Cell Growth

Investigators have strived to enhance vascular cell growth *in vitro*. SIMMS and STILLMAN [1937c] observed that the addition of trypsin to the nutrient caused 11-day-old fibroblasts from the chicken aorta to resume growth after 3 days of stagnancy. MORRISON *et al.* [1963] prepared several extracts from acetone-dried calf aortae and added these, or chondroitin sulfate A or B (CS-A, CS-B), for a 72-hour period to 7-day-old cultures of chicken aortic cells. The number of cells, and their dry weight, increased under the influence of an aortic extract (No. 1) and of CS-A. Additives stimulated cell division. Aortic glycoproteins are rich in aspartic acid and in glutamic acid which, according to SIMMS [1961], promote cell growth.

MURATA *et al.* [1965] resuspended 7-day-old chicken aortic cells at a 1:125 v/v ratio in MEM, added 0.2 μg/ml of H^3-uridine and H^3-thymidine in 5% calf serum, incubated the preparation, trypsinized and counted the cells. The uptake of uridine was greater by the second generation of cells (F^2) than by the first (F^1). Within 15 minutes, the label appeared in the nucleus; then in the perinuclear zone of the cytoplasm. Thymidine uptake by the nuclei, as checked by autoradiography, was the same in F^2 and F^1 cells. MURATA *et al.* [1966] used 0.2 μc/ml H^3-uridine or H^3-thymidine plus C^{14}-acetate 0.44 μc/ml of MEM. Incorporation rates became constant after 6 hours; nucleoprotein equilibrium was reached in 5 days, for each generation of cells. In F^1, incorporation increased from day to day; in F^2, it dropped after the 1st day.

Autoradiography was also used by CHOI *et al.* [1968] and by FLORENTIN *et al.* [1968, 1969] to follow the passage of H^3-thymidine into the DNA of minipig aortic cells exposed to normo- and hypercholesteremic serum. The incorporation of H^3-thymidine, pulsed for 30 minutes per day for 3 days against a mixed cell culture, was 31% on addition of hypercholesteremic serum, but only 22% when normocholesteremic serum was added to the nutrient. KAO *et al.* [1968] noted that on exposure to 5% hyperlipemic monkey serum the diameter of 14-day-old colonies of Rhesus aortic smooth muscle cells was 79 mm to 112 mm, compared with 25 mm of controls. CHOI *et al.* [1968] found that the incorporation of H^3-thymidine, C^{14}-leucine, and C^{14}-glycine for protein synthesis remained constant in surviving cells. The number of cells exposed to hypercholesteremic serum was 50% lower than in the controls. This numeric reduction of cells was ascribed to hypercholesteremia. However, it has long been known that rapid growth may expedite rapid degeneration and death of cells.

E. *Mixed Cell Populations*

1. Composition

A mixed cell population is established as soon as fibrocytes join the earlier-appearing endothelial cells and fat-laden cells. Such mixed populations persist until macrophages disintegrate and endothelial cells have disappeared. For rabbit aortic cells, this period has been fixed by POLLAK and KASAI [1964] as 10 to 12 days (fig. 9).

If the explant has been removed at an early date—as soon as the first outgrowth of cells appears—only fibrocytes will be present after the 12th day of the primary culture. If the explant is left *in situ*, fibrocytes will be joined by smooth muscle cells, at the time the other cells have vanished. A new mixed population develops, consisting of fibrocytes and myocytes. The proportion of the 2 cell types remains constant since they have comparable growth rates.

In a mixed culture, the growth of one cell type may be inhibited by the growth of another type. Endothelial cells and fibroblasts compete for nutrients, especially for certain amino acids. The 'hungrier' and more aggressive fibroblasts displace the delicate endothelial cells in the first mixed population. Fibrocytes and myocytes live in symbiosis, in the second mixed population. The density of the culture and the depletion of the nutrient are limiting factors.

In pure cultures, most cells will propagate continuously under stable conditions. This does not apply to macrophages loaded with lipoids.

2. Aging and Longevity of Cells

Endothelial cells begin to age shortly. They increase in size, stretch, and become distorted. The nuclei increase in size. Sometimes, the nuclei become bean or dumbbell shaped. Sometimes, binucleated cells develop when nuclear division is not followed by division of the cytoplasm. With aging, changes occur in the quantity of enzymes and in the distribution of enzymes within the cells. Aging cells lose cohesiveness and disperse easily. They lose adhesiveness and detach more readily from their support than younger cells (fig. 7).

Under favorable conditions, the birth rate of fibrocytes exceeds the death rate. The signs of fibrocytic aging are, to some extent, similar to those of

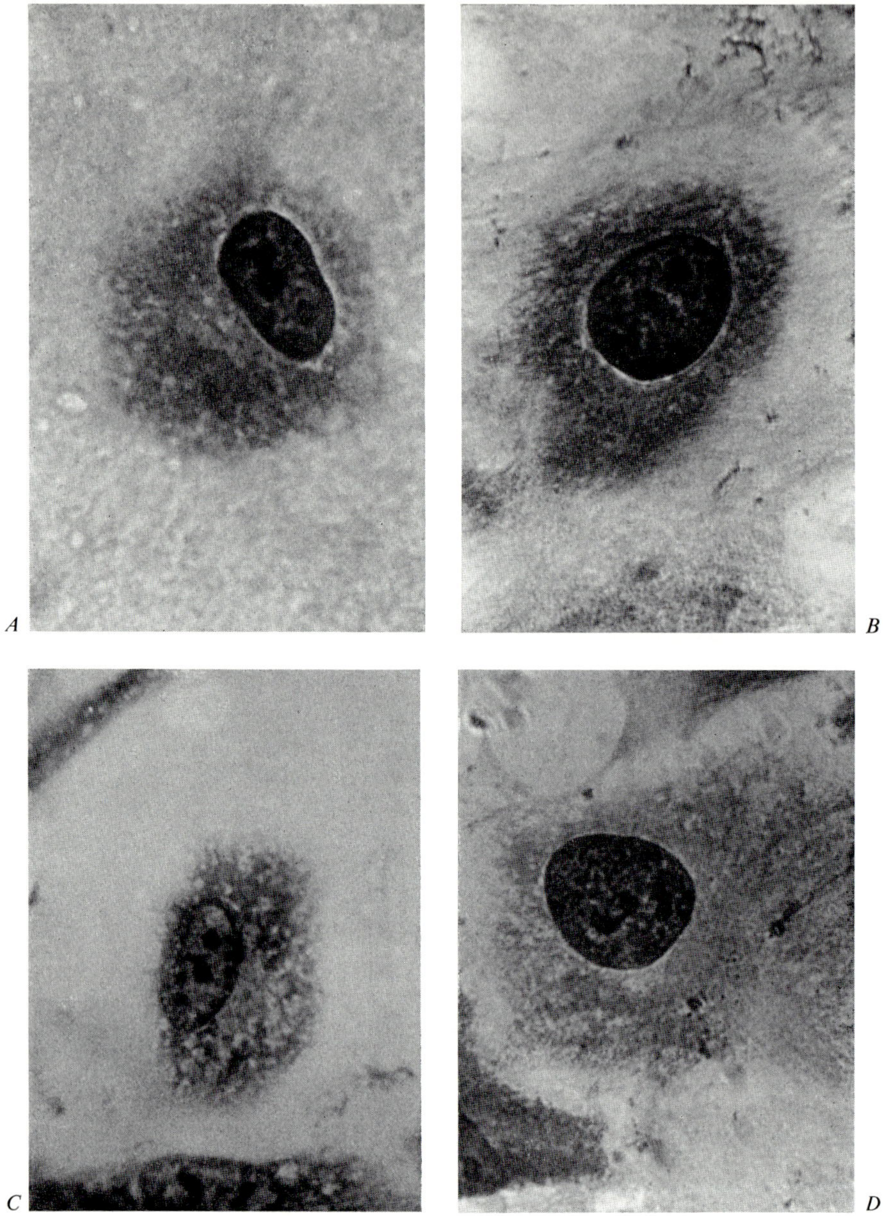

Fig. 7. Aging of aortic endothelial cells. *A.* Rabbit. Culture, 5 days old. *B.* Rabbit. Culture, 10 days old. *C.* Man. Culture, 6 days old. *D.* Man. Culture, 12 days old. May-Grünwald-Giemsa stain (×1000).

endothelial cells. Fibrocytes change from spindles to triangular, rhombohedric, and kite-like forms. This is due to stretching of the cells on the glass support. Spontaneous appearance of fat droplets is very characteristic. This must be taken into consideration by those who study lipoid metabolism of fibroblasts. Fat granules increase in number and in size after the 5th day. The cells shed these granules on about the 12th to 15th day (fig. 8). Loss of motility is another sign of aging. Enzyme changes, too, occur over time within the cells.

Nothing is known about the aging of vascular myocytes. Fat-laden macrophages do not age. As their motion ceases and the cells shed fat droplets, the cells disintegrate. LAZZARINI [1959] exposed *in vitro* endothelial cells for 72 to 96 hours to cholesterol suspensions (20 mg/ml). Cytolysis of such cells occurred 168 hours later.

The question of longevity is closely related to that of aging. In a mixed culture, human aortic cells live up to 14 days, according to BRANWOOD [1961a]. Rabbit aortic endothelial cells live up to 14 days, according to KOKUBU and POLLAK [1961c]; if the explant is left in place they can be seen after 4 weeks. LAZZARINI [1959] fixed the life span of fat-laden cells as 6 days. KOIDE *et al.* [1964] concurred, but occasionally observed these cells on the 10th day in cultures from rabbit aortae with experimentally induced plaques. When the explant has been kept *in situ*, fat-laden cells may be seen trapped between muscular syncytium. Fibrocytes and myocytes survive as long as favorable culture conditions are maintained. POLLAK and ADACHI [1968] followed these 2 cell types in cultures from rabbit aortae, human aortae, and smaller human arteries for 28 days.

3. Identification of Cells

Endothelail cells and fibrocytes *in vitro* can be easily identified under direct or under-phase contrast illumination, and in stained preparations. The experienced worker recognizes macrophages easily in unstained and in stained slides. To differentiate these cells from other cells which have become 'round', one must study their motility. The presence of smooth muscle cells is suspected whenever 2 crossing sheets or strands of elongated cells are seen. Identification of myocytes in unstained preparations is not reliable. FRITZ *et al.* [1969] could not distinguish myocytes from fibrocytes by light microscopic autoradiography with ^{3}H-thymidine. Of the many stains tried by KASAI and POLLAK [1964], Pollak's trichrome stain was the most satis-

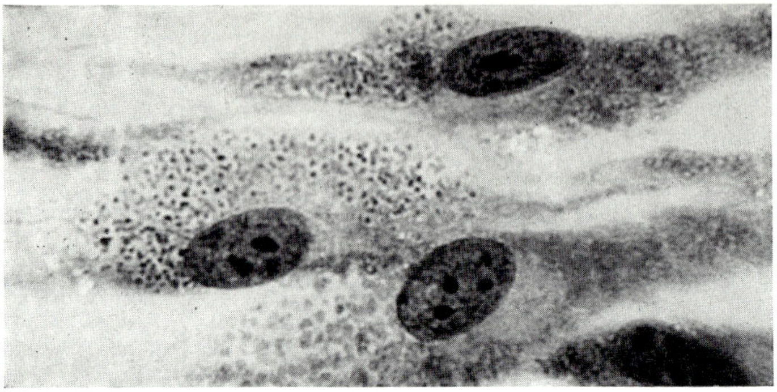

A

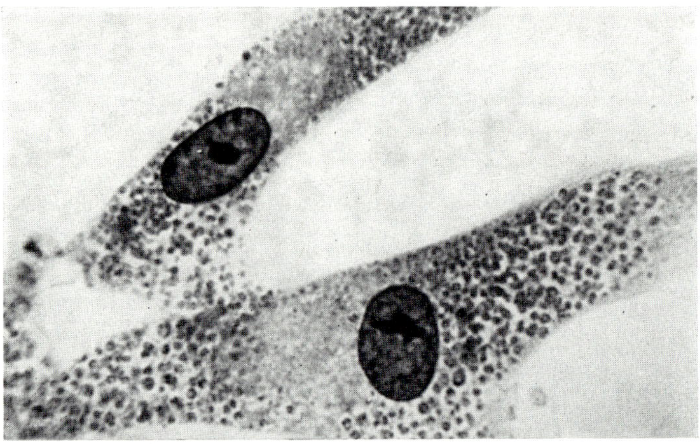

B

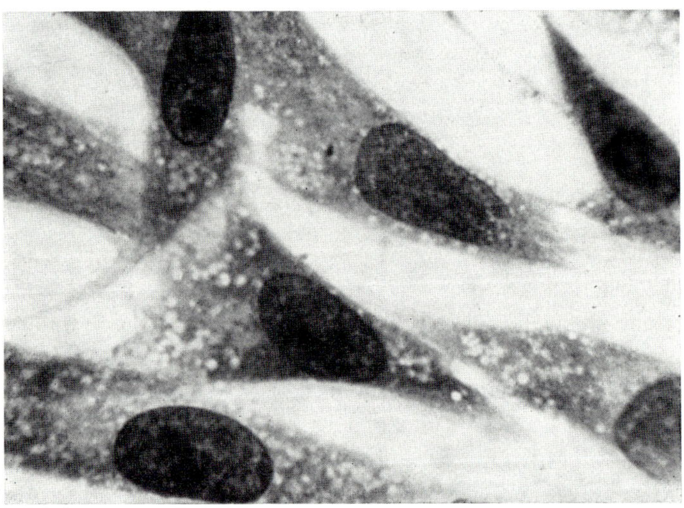

C

factory, since cytoplasmic myofilaments were demonstrated as delicate threads arranged parallel to the long axis of the muscle cells. KAO *et al.* [1968] identified aortic smooth muscle cells by staining with fluorescent actomycin globulin.

Cells can also be identified by more elaborate procedures. Cells differ in enzyme reactions, in phagocytic ability, in their susceptibility to viral infection, in resistance to toxins, and in the uptake of radioisotopes.

4. Isolation of Cells

Identification of cells is a prerequisite for cloning. For the cloning of endothelial cells, one has to select the earliest appearing cells, before the outgrowth of fibroblasts. SHIBUYA [1931], failing to obtain a pure culture of endothelial cells from chicken and rabbit aortae, suggested that an explant composed of a single cell type be used. Such an explant does not exist. BRANWOOD [1961a, 1963] used intimal endothelial pellicle explants. He obtained not only endothelial cells, but also fibroblasts. He suggested the use of a nutrient which would promote the growth of one particular cell type, or the addition of chemicals which would inhibit the growth of an undesired type. Blocking the mitosis of certain cells by x-ray irradiation is not useful. The removal of calcium and magnesium from the nutrient promotes loosening of cells. This is not practical. The only sensible method, at this time, is to use the micromanipulator to select cells for cloning.

In pure cultures, vascular endothelial cells and fibrocytes have been maintained for several generations. Isolation of myocytes has not been successful. Fat-laden macrophages can be isolated easily, but cannot be cloned.

SHIBUYA [1931] grew rabbit aortic cells for 4 generations. INGENITO *et al.* [1958] cultured human aortic fibroblasts for 3 generations and maintained them for up to 18 months. LAZZARINI [1961d] grew F^1–F^6 of human endothelial cells and fibroblasts within 2 weeks, and observed human and canine aortic cells for 8 weeks without noting significant changes in metabolic requirements [1962b]. AYKAN [1964] followed 22 generations of rat aortic

---

Fig. 8. Aging of rabbit aortic fibrocytes. *A.* Culture, 6 days old (normal granularity). *B.* Culture, 13 days old (increased granularity). *C.* Culture, 15 days old (degranulation). May-Grünwald-Giemsa stain (× 800).

fibroblasts for up to 175 days. He recorded that mitotic activity gradually decreased, and fatty degeneration gradually increased from the 4th passage of cells and from the 19th day on. ROBERTSON [1965a] studied cloned aortic cells from 10 weeks to 29 months, and he observed morphologic and chromosomal changes, giant cell formation, and metabolic variations. Chicken aortic endothelial cells were carried for 18 generations by MURATA *et al.* [1965, 1966, 1967]. They noted that the size of F^2 cells was larger than of F^1 cells, that the uptake of H^3 from labeled uridine was higher by F^2 cells than by F^1 cells, and that lipoid synthesis of F^3 cells exceeded that of F^2. Pigeon aortic cells were kept up to F^4 by SMITH *et al.* [1965]. CHOI *et al.* [1968b] obtained more than 15 generations of minipig aortic cells.

COOPER [1961] pointed out that the organ culture is the closest one to an *in vivo* environment, and that the primary cell culture is closer to *in vivo* conditions than the secondary or subsequent cultures. Cloned cells, out of contact with other cells, adapt more to the environment with each succeeding generation. The results of metabolic studies with cloned cells may lose, with each generation, validity for extrapolation to the *in vivo* situation.

One must bear in mind that the morphologic and the physiologic behavior of cells depend on the origin of the explant, the culture conditions, the generation, and the age of the cells in mixed or in pure cultures.

F. Endothelial Cells

1. Morphology

Analyzing cell descriptions and illustrations from vascular tissue culture literature, one must conclude that many early investigators failed to grow endothelial cells.

Omitting the negative and the doubtful reports, it appears that vascular endothelial cells were first obtained by SHIBUYA [1931] from rabbit aortae. PARSHLEY *et al.* [1953] described endothelial cells as cords or mosaics grown from dog, cat, goat, and human aortae. LAZZARINI [1959 and on] grew endothelial cells from the aortae and coronary arteries of man, chicken, dog,

---

Fig. 9. Mixed cell populations in primary cultures from rabbit aortae. *A.* From intact aorta (with endothelial cells and fibrocytes). *B.* From aorta with plaques (with endothelial cells, fibrocytes, and fat-laden macrophages). Cultures, 4 days old. Phase contrast, stop-motion, cinephotomicrography (× 160).

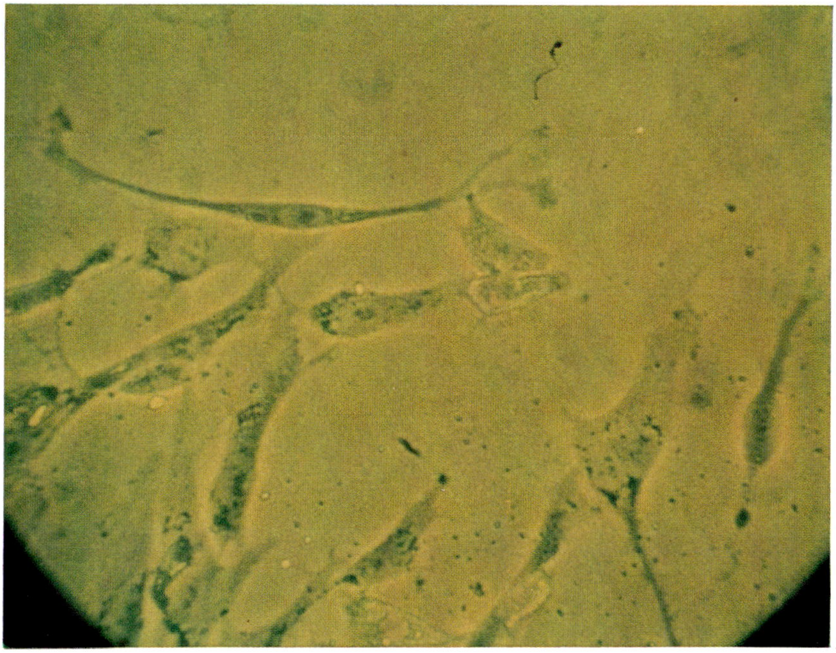

9 A

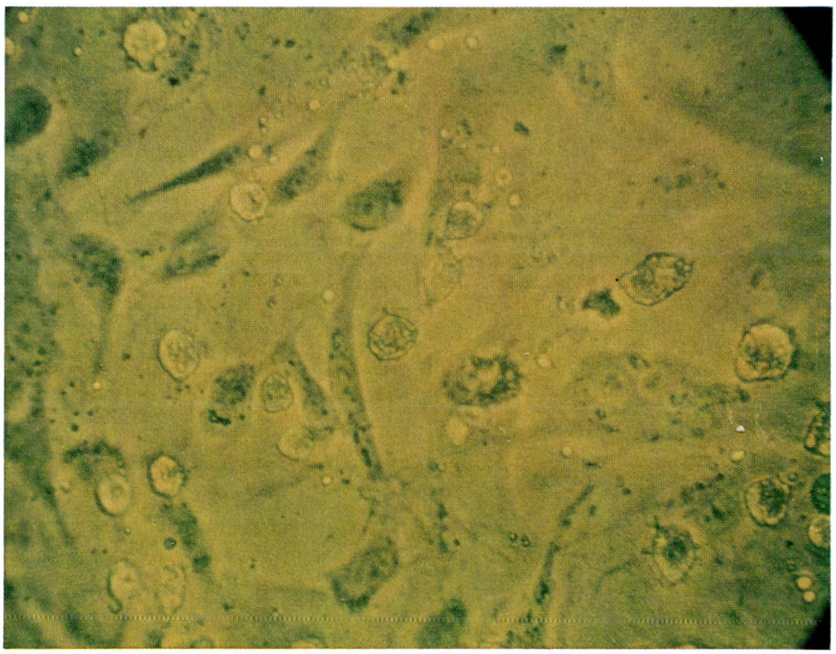

9 B

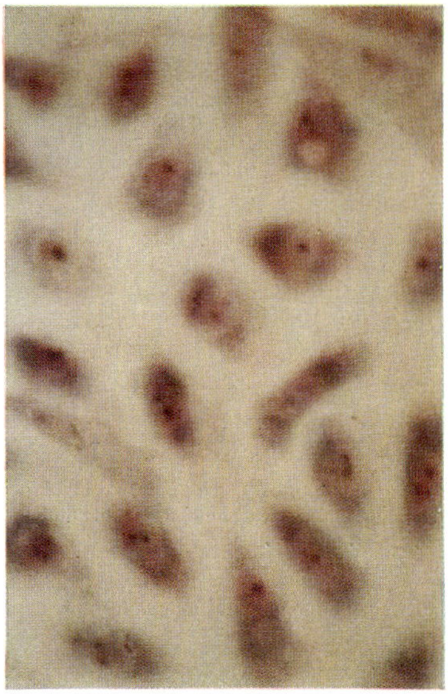

10 A

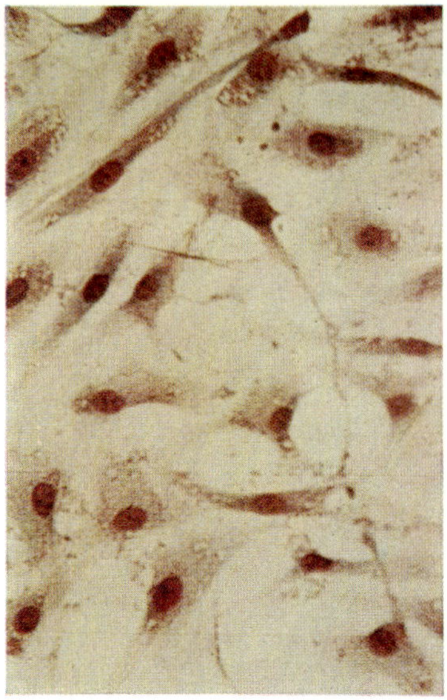

10 B

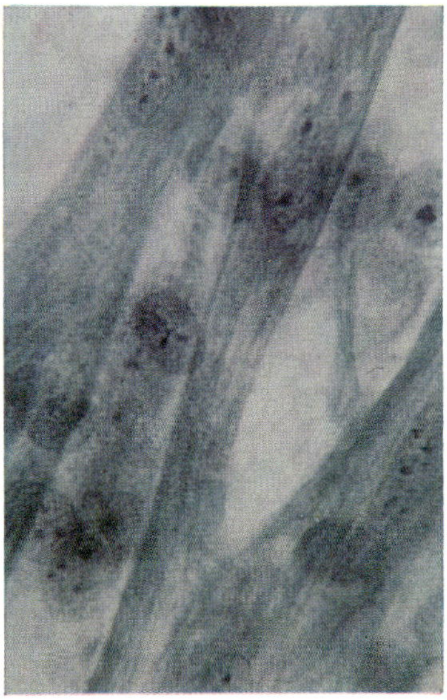

10 C

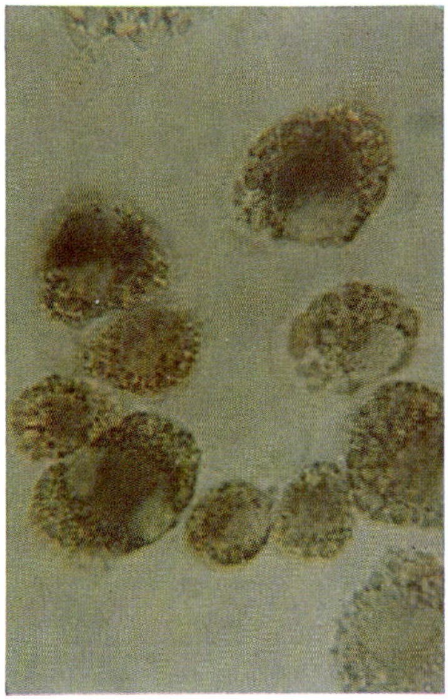

10 D

Table V. Morphologic characteristics of rabbit aortic endothelial cells

Size	30 μ × 40 μ; older cells, up to 70 μ × 120 μ
Shape	'round'—polygonal
Profile	flying saucer-like
Nucleus	1 central or paracentral; 20 μ × 20 μ; abnormally, 2 nuclei
Nucleoli	2 or 4, poorly visible
Golgi zone	narrow, perinuclear
Mitochondria	many
Ribosomes	abundant
Granules	few, small; older cells, more and larger
Cytoplasm	homogeneous; a reticular, dense inner zone; a translucent outer zone; pynocytic vesicles at cell membrane
Protrusions	none; membrane-like periphery

mouse, and rabbit. BRANWOOD [1951a, 1963] cultured endothelial cells from human aortic intima, KOKUBU and POLLAK [1961b and on] from the aortae of rabbits, and POLLAK *et al.* [1962a and on] from human arteries. MORRISON *et al.* [1963] and MURATA *et al.* [1965 and on] grew endothelial cells from chicken aortae, MURATA [1968] from the aorta of rhesus monkeys, and CHOI *et al.* [1968] from the aortae of minipigs.

The most detailed morphologic description of endothelial cells was presented by KOIDE *et al.* [1963] and KASAI *et al.* [1964] for rabbit aortic cells, and by POLLAK and ADACHI [1968] for human arterial cells. The latter found that human cells differ from rabbit cells only slightly: The nuclei of human cells contain less chromatin and stain lighter. The description of human endothelial cells rendered by LAZZARINI [1959, 1963a], and by ROBERTSON [1965a] for 'intimacytes' also matched that given by KASAI *et al.* [1964] for rabbit cells (table V).

No significant disparities in the morphologic appearance of vascular endothelial cells from different species, sites, and donor ages were noted by

Fig. 10. Pure cultures of rabbit aortic cells. *A.* Endothelial cells. Culture, 6 days old. Giemsa stain (×160). *B.* Fibrocytes. Culture, 6 days old. Giemsa stain (×160). *C.* Myocytes. Culture, 14 days old. Pollak's trichrome stain (×500). *D.* Fat-laden macrophages. Culture, 3 days old. Esterase stain (×450). [Figure 10C is figures 30–13 in POLLAK, O.J., 1965; reproduced with permission of Hoeber Medical Division, Harper and Row, New York.]

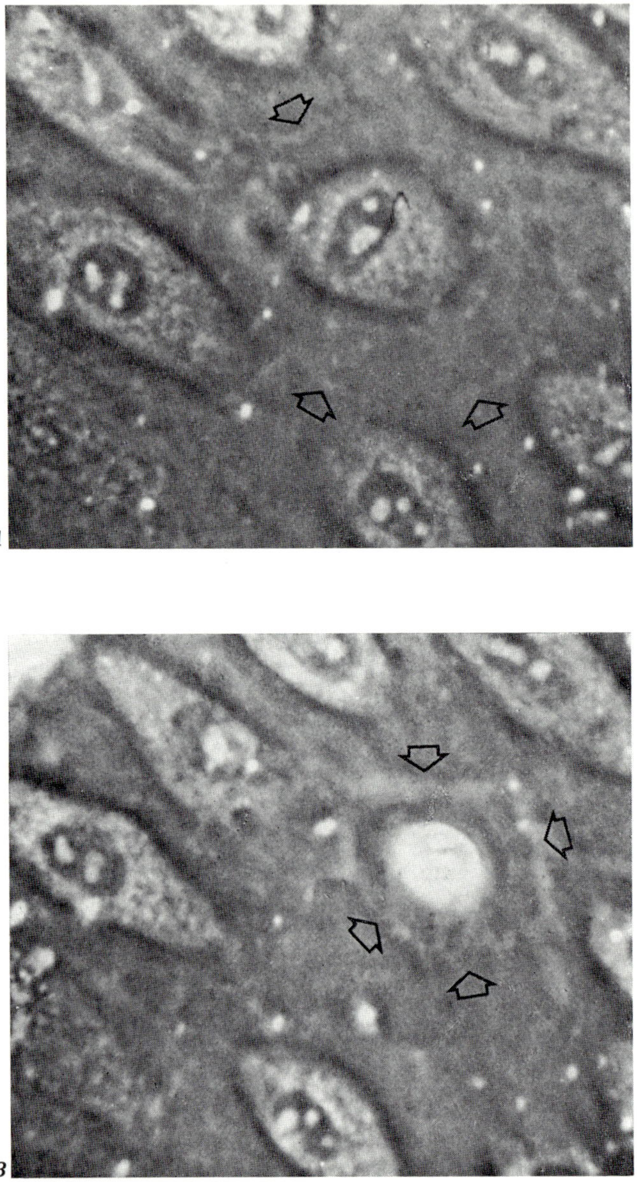

A

B

Fig. 11. Rabbit aortic endothelial cells. *A*. Before mitosis. *B*. During mitosis (reflecting light). (Arrows indicate cell borders.) Phase contrast; time-lapse cinephotomicrography (×400). [Figures 7 and 8 in POLLAK, O.J. and KASAI, T., 1964; reproduced with permission of Lea and Febiger, Philadelphia.]

POLLAK and ADACHI [1968], who compared rabbit aortic cells with cells from the aortae and smaller arteries of men of differing ages.

A pure endothelial cell monolayer culture is characterized by uniformity of the cells (fig. 10A).

2. Biology

a) Kinetics

The only references to the movement of endothelial cells were made by KASAI *et al.* [1964] and POLLAK and KASAI [1964]. They were recorded in a motion picture by POLLAK and BURNS [1965]. Endothelial cells from rabbit aortae move in amoeba-like fashion away from the explant to the periphery. Their Brownian movement is sluggish and it speeds-up only during the process of cell division.

b) Reproduction

The possibility of amitotic cell division was considered by KOIDE *et al.* [1963] as they observed endothelial cells with bean-shaped or dumbbell-shaped nuclei. However, as a rule, endothelial cells propagate by mitosis. KASAI *et al.* [1964] followed 30 aortic endothelial cells for 7 hours under time lapse cinephotomicrography and observed that 7 cells underwent mitosis during this period. The total mitotic cycle lasted from 20 to 30 minutes (fig. 3). During mitosis, the cells became spheric and reflected the light (fig. 11).

G. Fibrocytes – Fibroblasts

1. Morphology

All the researchers who have attempted vascular tissue cultures have obtained spindle cells, alone or together with endothelial cells. Most authors refer to these cells as 'fibroblasts' although this is an incorrect designation. PARSHLEY *et al.* [1953] described fibroblasts grown from aortae of many species, as did LAZZARINI [1959]. ROBERTSON [1965a] compared 'fibrophils' with 'intimacytes' of human aortic cultures. All descriptions of fibroblasts come close to the detailed accounts, made by KOIDE *et al.* [1963], and KASAI and POLLAK [1964], for cells from rabbit aortae, and those by POLLAK and ADACHI [1968] for human aortae and other arteries. In the latter report, it was pointed out that human fibroblasts are somewhat broader, 20 μ to 30 μ against 10 μ to 15 μ, and that the nuclear membrane of human fibroblasts

Table VI. Morphologic characteristics of rabbit aortic fibrocytes

Size	10 μ to 15 μ × 18 μ to 120 μ; older cells, 30 μ to 40 μ × 80 μ to 120 μ
Shape	spindle; older cells, triangular, rectangular, polygonal, kite-like
Profile	spindle shaped or slender rhomboid
Nucleus	1 central, oval, broad, with a thick membrane
Nucleoli	2 to 4, clearly visible, distinct, regular
Golgi zone	distinct, to 1 pole of the nucleus
Mitochondria	scattered
Granules	many, small; older cells, more and coarse, less uniformly sized; still older cells, fewer. Pink (Giemsa's stain, PAS stain), green (Pollak's stain), dark under phase illumination
Cytoplasm	homogeneous; later, coarse, few pinocytic vesicles. Light blue (Giemsa's stain), greenish (Pollak's stain)
Protrusions	2, slender, fibrillar, up to 75 μ long; later, shorter, often split in swallow-tail fashion

is not quite as thick as that of rabbit cells. Age and sex apparently had no influence on the appearance of arterial fibroblasts. WEXLER and THOMAS [1967] used male rats and female virgins, or breeder rats who had had 4 or more pregnancies as donors for aortic cultures. They did not comment on cell morphology. KASAI and POLLAK [1964] found that aortic fibroblasts are slightly larger, and have larger nuclei, than fibroblasts from tendons of the same rabbit (table VI).

The pleomorphism of fibrocytes in pure monolayer culture is prominent (fig. 10B).

2. Biology

a) Kinetics

As fibrocytes migrate from the explant, they remain connected end-to-end for some time. POLLAK and BURNS [1965] followed the motion of fibrocytes by cinephotomicrography. Young fibrocytes have an active, gliding movement. Their bodies curve slightly during forward movement. They do not travel in a straight line but in an oblique, avoiding other cells and particles. With aging, the motion becomes slower.

Fig. 12. A. Syncytial growth of rabbit aortic myocytes. Culture, 18 days old. Pollak's trichrome stain (× 1050). *B.* Mitosis in a rabbit aortic myocyte. Culture, 18 days old. Pollak's trichrome stain (× 1050).

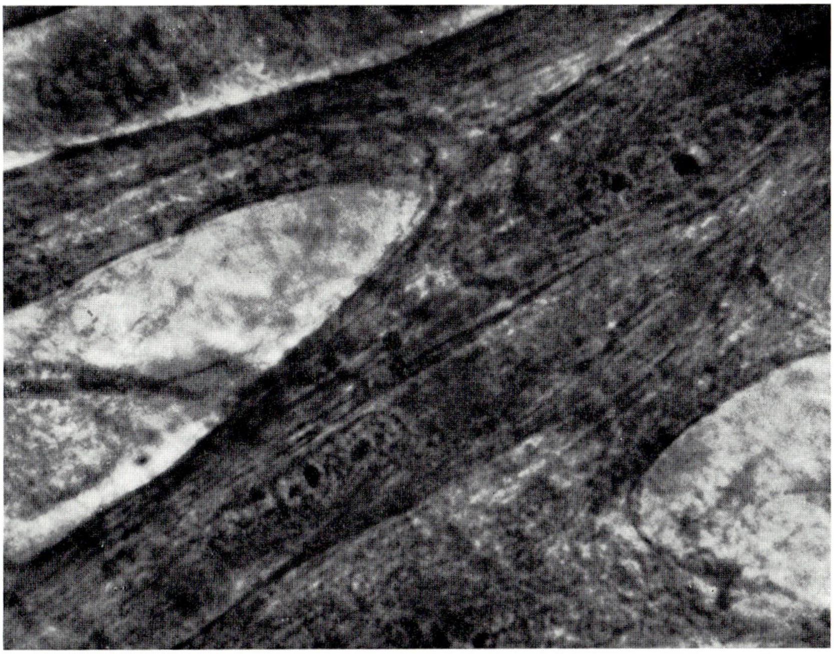

A

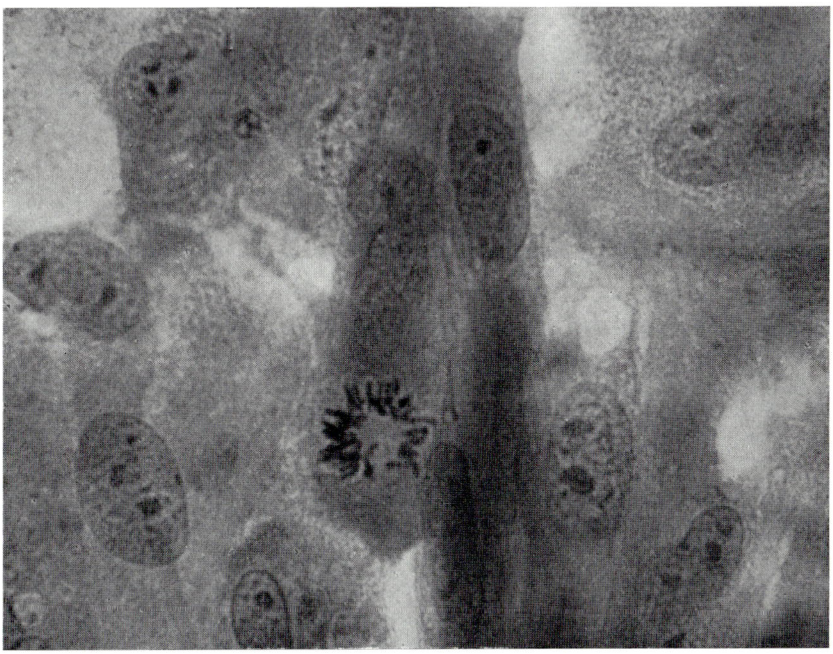

B

b) Reproduction

Fibroblasts propagate by mitosis. According to KOIDE *et al.* [1963] it takes 15 to 20 minutes for a spindle cell to become 'round' and another 15 to 20 minutes for the formation and separation of 2 new spindle cells (fig. 3).

H. Myocytes – Smooth Muscle Cells

1. Morphology

There are few reports on vascular smooth muscle cells in tissue culture literature. This is because explants have generally been removed as soon as the first cells appeared. The description of 4% of cells seen by PARSHLEY *et al.* [1953] in a few 6½-week-old canine aortic cultures leaves no doubt that these were smooth muscle cells. WEXLER and THOMAS [1967] mentioned the presence of smooth muscle cells in rat aortic cultures. Using the mid-portion of the aortic wall as explant, KAO *et al.* [1968] grew smooth muscle cells from Rhesus monkeys. A detailed description of smooth muscle cells from rabbit aortae came from KASAI and POLLAK [1964a] (fig. 10C). POLLAK and ADACHI [1968] stated that myocytes from human aortae and smaller arteries could not be distinguished morphologically from rabbit aortic muscle cells. KASAI and POLLAK [1964a] noted that muscle cells grown from atherosclerotic aortic segments were larger and broader than muscle cells from intact segments of rabbit aortae (table VII).

2. Biology

a) Kinetics

Vascular smooth muscle cells migrate toward the periphery of the preparation. They spread in a syncytial fashion, and no isolated cells can be seen (fig. 12A). Thus, the length of the cells can only be estimated. The cells tend to form a dense, curved, central cord, from which new cells spread in radiating fashion (fig. 5B). True motion of vascular myocytes has not been observed by KASAI *et al.* [1964].

b) Reproduction

Smooth muscle cells reproduce by mitosis (fig. 12B). The complete mitotic cycle has not been followed, however, because identification of these cells in unstained preparation is difficult. Observation under cinephotomicro-

Table VII. Morphologic characteristics of rabbit aortic myocytes

Size	20 μ × 160 μ (?)
Shape	ribbon-like
Profile	cylindric
Nucleus	1 oval, large, slender, 8 μ to 10 μ × 25 μ to 30 μ, with a thin membrane
Nucleoli	1 to 3, mostly indistinct
Golgi zone	indistinct
Myofilaments	many, slender, parallel to long axis. Pink (Giemsa's stain), black (Pollak's stain)
Cytoplasm	homogeneous. Pink (Giemsa's stain), grayish (Pollak's stain)
Protrusions	none

graphy is hampered by the fact that smooth muscle cells form an interwoven network with the arterial fibroblasts (fig. 6). The culture technic of KAO *et al.* [1968] may lead to isolation of aortic smooth muscle cells in pure cultures which could be utilized for studies not yet performed.

I. Fat-laden Macrophages

The origin of fat-laden cells characteristic of atherosclerosis has been often discussed. Different cells have been singled out as the precursors of cells which in stained preparations present as 'foam cells'. The endothelial cell has often been selected as the mother cell, the myocyte, the fibrocyte, and the tissue mast cell—which has not yet been seen in vascular tissue cultures, although its presence in the intima-subintima has been proven. Reticulo-endothelial cells and most circulating blood cells have been mentioned as precursors of 'foam cells'. Since such cells isolated *in vitro* from atherosclerotic aortae of rabbits and of man are indistinguishable from fat-laden macrophages of the abdominal cavity one could assume that one or more cell types can transform into macrophages before or during the process of cellular lipoidosis.

1. Morphology

The conversion of human intimal cells into fat-laden cells upon exposure to hyperlipemic serum was reported by BRANWOOD [1961a, 1963]. LAZZARINI [1959] referred to transformation of endothelial cells into 'foam cells' within 72 hours of incubation in a nutrient containing 20 mg/ml cholesterol. Fat droplets, 0.5 μ to 2 μ, appeared, and increased in size with further incubation until, at 168 hours, the cells had 2 to 3 large vacuoles and underwent cytolysis. LAZZARINI [1961d, 1962b] repeated this experiment with lipoprotein. Treated cells had a strong positive Lieberman-Burchard reaction to cholesterol and reacted to Sudan IV and Sudan Black B. ROBERTSON [1967b] converted 'intimacytes' into 'atherophils' through exposure to aqueous cholesterol suspensions.

While much attention was being paid to lipoid incorporation, none was paid to cell morphology. An informative description was rendered by DAY *et al.* [1966], who separated fat-laden macrophages from rabbit aortic plaques for study of phospholipoid synthesis by these cells.

There is no doubt that the 'round' cells from canine grafts, described by PARSHLEY *et al.* [1953], were fat-laden macrophages. KOKUBU [1961 and on] reported small round cells cultured from explants of rabbit aortae with plaques, but he failed to identify them properly. He called them 'modified endothelial cells' (IIIb), differing from normal endothelial cells (IIIa). KASAI *et al.* [1964], POLLAK and KASAI [1964], and POLLAK and BURNS [1965], using cinephotomicrography combined with the reverse phase contrast and with the stop-motion technic, established the identity of these cells. The cells matched peritoneal macrophages with lipoid content, in all respects (fig. 10D). According to POLLAK and ADACHI [1968] human fat-laden macrophages are smaller than corresponding cells from rabbits; the cytoplasm of human cells is less coarse and human cells have fewer projections (table VIII).

Fat-laden macrophages from one explant represent a fairly uniform population, except for some variation in size; cells from different explants are pleomorphic (fig. 13).

Table VIII. Morphologic characteristics of rabbit aortic fat-laden macrophages

Size	20 μ × 20 μ to 40 μ × 40 μ
Shape	round
Profile	spheric, burr-like
Nucleus	1 large, round, central, 16 μ × 16 μ to 30 μ × 30 μ
Nucleoli	1
Golgi zone	narrow, perinuclear, indistinct
Granules	many, coarse, scattered
Cytoplasm	neutrophilic or acidophilic
Protrusions	many, short, spike- or thorn-like; or, pseudopodia, tentacles

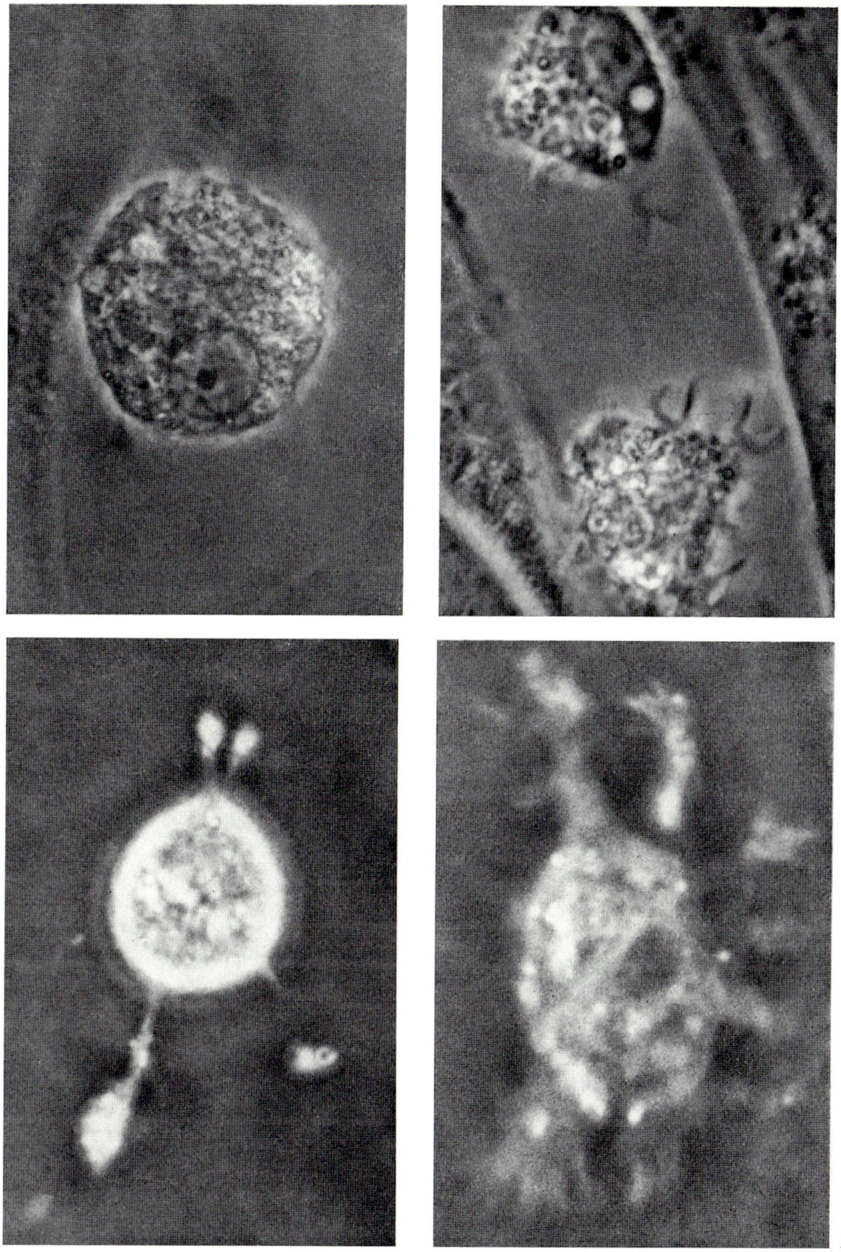

A B C D

Fig. 13. A–D. Pleomorphism of fat-laden macrophages from rabbit aortic plaques. Cultures, 1–2 days old. Reverse phase contrast (×1000–×1200). [Figure 13D is figure 4 in KASAI, T.; POLLAK, O.J. and NAGASAWA, S., 1964; reproduced with permission of Springer, Berlin/Göttingen/Heidelberg.]

2. Biology

a) Kinetics

The movements of fat-laden macrophages were monitored by Kasai *et al.* [1964] and Pollak and Burns [1965]. In contrast to endothelial cells, these cells have a permanent luminescence (fig. 13). Since these cells do not grow or reproduce, one cannot speak of an outgrowth from the explant or of a cell culture. Fat-laden macrophages simply separate from the explant. Because of their rapid, meteorite-like movement they are seen throughout the preparation.

b) Reproduction

Those who have experimentally transformed endothelial cells into 'foam cells'—Branwood [1963], Lazzarini [1961d, 1962b], and Robertson [1967]—have found that these cells do not propagate. In spite of continuous observation for 3 days, Kasai *et al.* [1964] and Pollak and Burns [1965] failed to record any multiplication of fat-laden macrophages. Tume *et al.* [1969] isolated 'foam cells' from rabbit aorta but failed in their attempts to grow these cells on fibroblasts feeder layers. Thus, it may be concluded that the fat-laden cell, regardless of origin, is incapable of reproduction.

J. Lipoid Transport by Cells in vitro

Much work has been devoted to the study of the transport of lipoids by nonvascular and by vascular cells. Studies on the cellular level seem especially important because the formation of fat-laden cells, which are so characteristic of early spontaneous and experimental atherogenesis, is still a subject of speculation. Pinocytosis, phagocytosis, and simple transfer mediated by lipfanogens have been considered.

1. Pinocytosis

Pinocytosis takes place on the cell membrane. Microvilli—pinocytic vesicles—were described in vascular cells, namely in endothelial cells, by Lazzarini [1959, 1960a, 1960b] who ascribed an active role in lipoid trans-

Fig. 14. A. Spontaneous sudanophilia of rabbit aortic cells. Culture, 30 days old. Sudan black B (×260). *B.* Experimental sudanophilia of rabbit aortic cells upon 3-day incubation in nutrient with cholesterol (2 mg/1 ml). Sudan black B (×260).

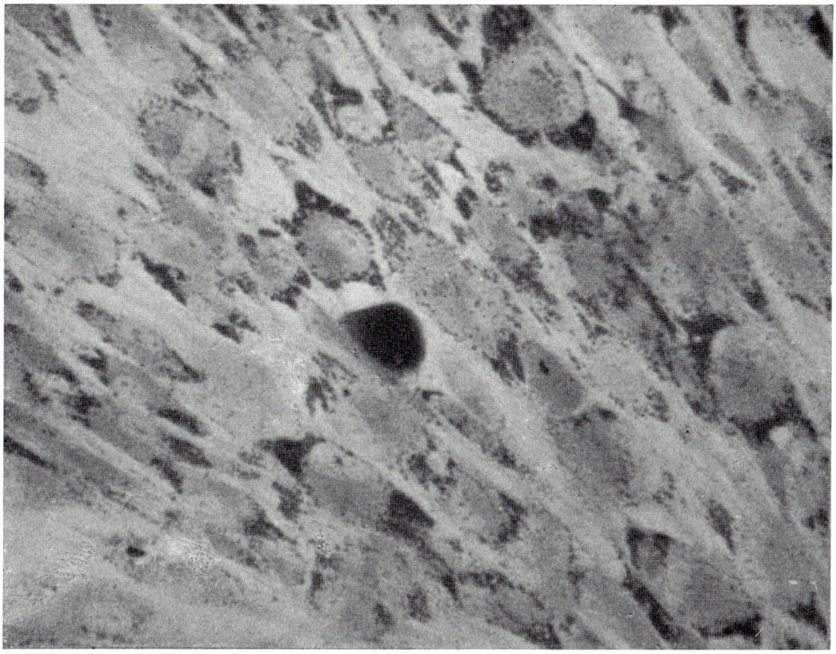

A

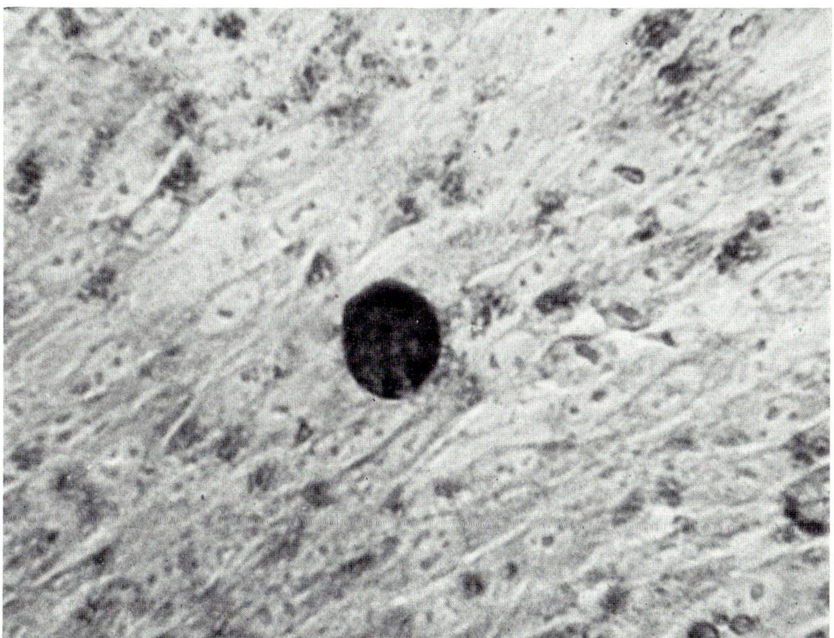

B

port to pinocytes. However, LAZZARINI [1961b] found that the addition of ferritin, colloidal gold, or saccharide iron oxide modified the lipoid deposit in endothelial cells when microemulsions of radioactively labeled cholesterol were added to the nutrient. Instead of making reference to pinocytosis, he attributed the lipoid deposit to active competitive phagocytosis by endothelial cells.

2. Phagocytosis

Phagocytosis, the active engulfment of particles by cells, was studied by LAZZARINI [1959]. He added carbon particles (250 Å), 10 mg/ml, and saccharated iron oxide, 100 μg/ml, to nutrient. The material was incorporated into endothelial cells but not into fibroblasts of human aortae. Incubation of cells with 50 mg/ml cholesterol for 96 hours before a 10-day incubation with 20 μg of carbon resulted in the deposit of cholesterol but not of carbon. Pinocytosis was considered to be insignificant by LAZZARINI [1962a]. ROBERTSON [1965b] stated that lipoid transport into endothelial cells is by phagocytosis rather than by pinocytosis.

The phagocytic potential of rabbit aortic endothelial cells and fibroblasts was studied in mixed and in pure cultures, by KOIDE and POLLAK [1962], and by POLLAK *et al.* [1962b]. Cells from normal and atherosclerotic sectors were used. The evaluation of the incorporation of nonradioactive particles was greatly hampered, and the results discredited, because of spontaneous increase in the number and size of cytoplasmic lipoid granules in aging cells, especially in fibroblasts. The amount of spontaneously accumulated sudanophilic material in a 1-month-old culture (fig. 14A) was found to exceed that in a 1-week-old culture which had been incubated for 3 days in a nutrient containing 20 mg cholesterol per ml (fig. 14B).

KOIDE and POLLAK [1962] prepared suspensions of lithium carmine of 1 μ to 3 μ particle size in lieu of cholesterol suspensions. They added 8×10^7 particles per ml of nutrient. The number of particles was adjusted to 10, 25, 50, 100, 200, and 400 per cell, before incubation. Cells were counted in aliquots of suspension cultures hourly for 6 hours/37 °C. The percentage of cells with carmine and the number of cells with more than 5 particles was counted in slides fixed in cold buffered formalin 10% and stained with Methylene Blue. Endothelial cells were 3 times as active as fibroblasts during the first 2 hours. It was in this period that greater activity was observed among cells from aortic plaques. Macrophages were packed with dye (fig. 15A).

Upon trypsinization of 17-day-old cultures and transfer from suspension culture to monolayer culture, phagocytosis of endothelial cells decreased while that of fibroblasts increased. KASAI and POLLAK [1964] ascribed this to the change in culture conditions. In another series, cells were first incubated with either (a) normocholesteremic rabbit serum (60 mg cholesterol/100 ml), (b) hypercholesteremic rabbit serum (800 mg/100 ml), or (c) a cholesterol suspension with 1 μ particle size. Next, cells were incubated with carmine suspension, 1 μ to 3 μ particles. There was no statistical difference in phagocytic activity in the 4 series (the 4th being a carmine control). No competitive or selective phagocytosis was observed. The particle size played no role in the experiments.

Until recently, the phagocytic potential of nonvascular and especially of vascular endothelial cells has been denied or underestimated. This opinion has now been corrected (fig. 15B).

A reduction of fat granules in the transformed endothelial cells occurred upon addition of 5% dialyzed human serum albumin to the culture media with human aortic cells, according to LAZZARINI [1959]. No systematic attempts have been made to influence vascular cell phagocytosis by physiologic means, such as by the addition of hormones, or through medication.

3. Lipfanogens and Antilipfanogen

Since phagocytosis requires freedom of movement for the cells, which actively engulf foreign matter, it is questionable whether the process, which can be so readily demonstrated *in vitro*, actually takes place *in vivo*. The migrant smooth muscle cell, which in the process of atherogenesis penetrates the subintima from the muscular layer of the arterial wall, may be more capable of phagocytosis than stationary cells. Regrettably, the phagocytic potential of arterial smooth muscle cells has not been studied.

The passage of lipoids through the cell membrane into the cytoplasm seems a likely mechanism by which lipoids enter the cell. SIMMS [1936] and SIMMS *et al.* [1947] identified the serum 'B' factor which produces cellular lipoidosis and is now known as 'lipfanogens', substances consisting of soluble lipoids which become converted into visible granules. Such phanerosis is blocked by the antilipfanogen present in Cohn's serum albumin V fraction. Enzyme-activated precursors can be converted into additional lipfanogens by 2 to 3 days of incubation of serum at 37°C. Cytoplasmic fat granules may form as the result from the failure of cells to block the entry of lipfanogens, or by the failure to metabolize entered lipoids. Antilipfanogen either prevents the entry of lipoids, or enhances their metabolism after entry. Free lipfanogens are taken up by cells, whereas lipfanogens combined with antilipfanogen are not. This concept was supported by experimentation with adult chicken fibroblasts *in vitro* exposed to various blood sera and serum fractions. SIMMS *et al.* [1947] assayed the 3 fractions, lipfanogens, lipfanogen precursors, and antilipfanogen. They observed marked species differences with regard to the amounts of these 3 substances in serum. SIMMS and HARMISON [1966] claimed a correlation between lipfanogen/antilipfanogen ratios and the prevalence of atherosclerosis.

The fixation of free antilipfanogens by hypercholesteremic serum from patients with diabetes mellitus and from patients with clinical atherosclerosis was reported by LEWIS [1961]. Lipfanogen/antilipfanogen ratios of 1.63 and 1.58 were obtained for male and female patients, compared with 0.63 and 0.60 ratios for healthy men and women, respectively. GEER [1961] proposed that patients with clinical atherosclerosis have an advanced degree of atherogenesis with combined and complicated lesions. He suggested that the lipfanogen concept may explain the initiation of lipoid plaques, but not the evolution of fibrous and calcified lesions. One may argue that atherogenesis is an episodic process. 'Early' fatty lesions may develop in the presence of advanced lesions. Thus, an altered lipfanogen/antilipfanogen ratio may be indicative of a new crop of fatty plaques. The origin of lipoids found in various stages of atherogenesis may not always be the same. Initially, most lipoids are of exogenous origin; in later stages, endogenous local lipogenesis plays a greater role.

K. Metabolism

1. General Comments

Until now, most studies have revolved around lipoid metabolism, while a few have dealt with mucopolysaccharides. Amino acids have been only studied superficially. Nothing is known about the turnover of carbohydrates, minerals, and trace elements by vascular cells.

Fig. 15. A. Phagocytosis of carmine particles (1 μ) by 4 macrophages (dark, round), 1 endothelial cell (at right edge) and several fibrocytes from rabbit aortic plaque. Culture, 5 days old. Methylene Blue stain (×200). *B.* Phagocytosis by a rabbit aortic endothelial cell (in center). Culture, 26 hours old. Stop-motion, cinephotomicrography (×160).

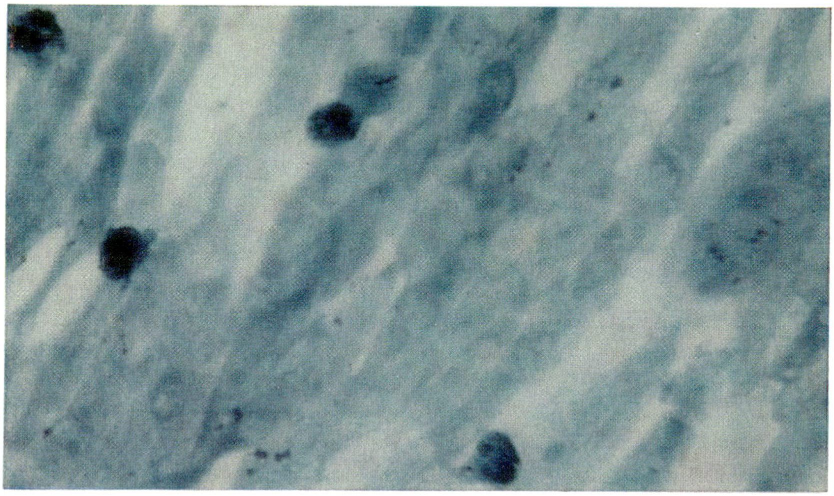

15 A

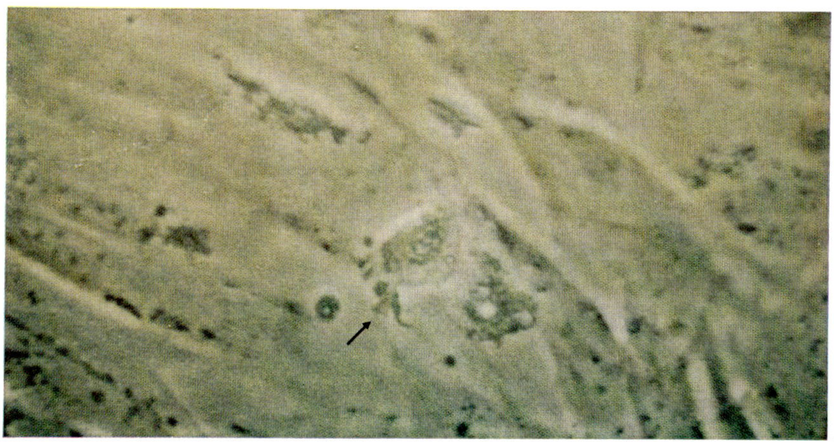

15 B

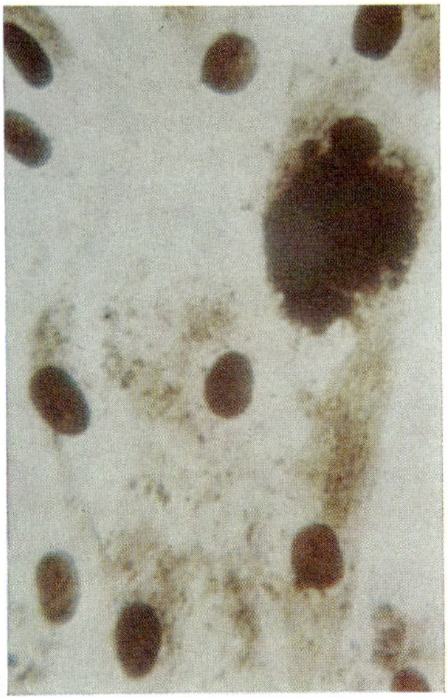

16 A

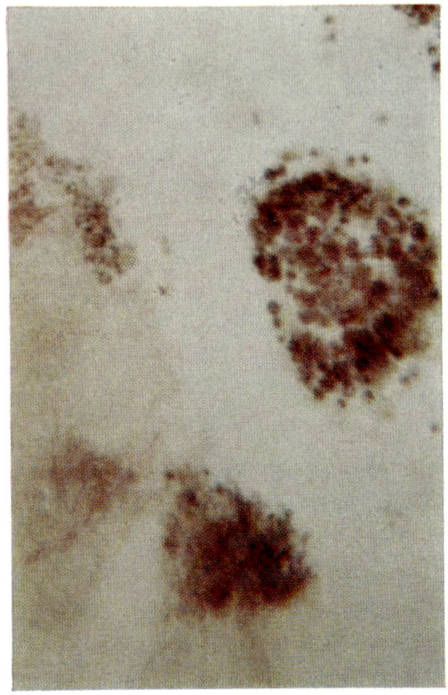

16 B

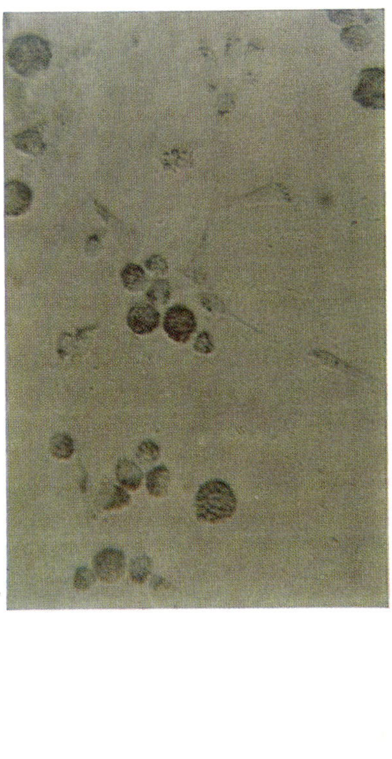

16 C

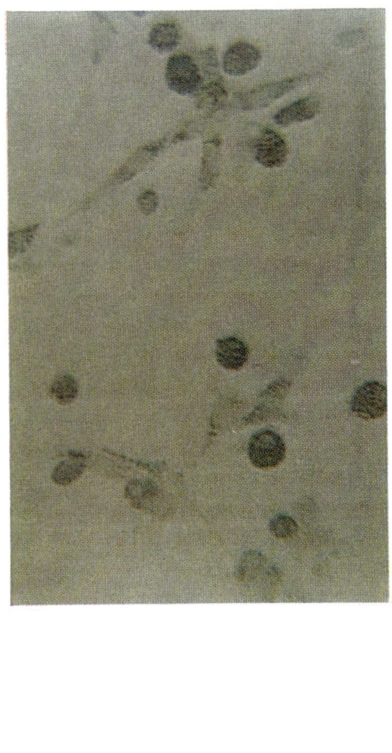

16 D

The preceding paragraph discloses the gaps in our knowledge about vascular cell metabolism and points to the complexity of the whole problem. Every facet of cell metabolism can be studied in multiple ways. One can use mixed cell populations, pure cell lines, young cells, old cells, cells from intact and altered tissues, cells from different species, from young and old subjects, cells from various anatomic sites, and cells grown under different conditions. Chemical analysis of the nutrient can and should be matched against chemical and cytochemical studies of the cells themselves.

2. Enzymes

In atherosclerosis research, arterial enzymes have been studied by histochemistry and by chemical analysis of tissues. Difficulties in comparing the results of these studies are due to the fact that different material has been assayed by a variety of techniques.

There is a sharp contrast between the comprehensive bibliography on enzyme studies of whole arteries and the scantiness of information on the enzymatic activity of vascular cells. There has been no analysis of cells. Some data are available on cytochemical studies, but are plagued by a lack of information as to methodology and by the fact that different methods, yielding different results, have been used.

KOIDE and POLLAK [1963a] applied 2 methods for acid phosphatase (pH 5.2) to cells grown from the same explant of rabbit atherosclerotic aorta. Macrophages had strongly, uniformly stained nuclei, and a weakly stained perinuclear zone; endothelial cells and fibrocytes had weakly stained nuclei and a faintly stained cytoplasm, when Gomori's method was used (fig. 16A). Using the azo-dye coupling method of Pearse, macrophages stained heavily in a coarse-granular manner; the nuclei of endothelial cells and fibrocytes did not stain at all, the juxtanuclear cytoplasm reacted slightly (fig. 16B).

LAZZARINI [1959] found normal endothelial cells strongly positive for succinic dehydrogenase, while cells with lipoid were weakly positive. Ac-

---

Fig. 16. A and *B*. Rabbit aortic cells stained for acid phosphatase (pH 5.2). Culture, 5 days old (large cells, macrophages) (×1000). *A*. Gomori's stain. *B*. Pearse's stain. *C* and *D*. Rabbit aortic cells from plaque stained for: *C*. succinic dehydrogenase by Scarpelli-Pearse's stain; *D*. for carboxyl esterase by Pearse's stain. Culture, 5 days old (round cells, macrophages) (×40).

cording to LAZZARINI [1961b, 1963a] endothelial cells stained positive for acid phosphatase, for enzymes of the citric acid cycle, for choline esterase, and for catepsin activity. The latter reaction increased considerably when 'intimacytes' were converted into 'atherophiles' by ROBERTSON [1965a].

Endothelial cells grown from rabbit aortae were found to be negative for alkaline phosphatase and adenosine triphosphatase, and weakly positive for acid phosphatase and succinic dehydrogenase by KOIDE and POLLAK [1963]. Fibrocytes gave similar reactions. KASAI and POLLAK [1964] obtained weakly positive reactions for alkaline phosphatase and adenosine triphosphatase in fat-laden macrophages, fairly strong reactions for acid phosphatase, for cytochrome oxidase C, succinic dehydrogenase (fig. 16C), and carboxyl esterase (fig. 16D). The stronger reaction for succinic dehydrogenase in fat-laden cells, compared with endothelial cells, contrasted with the findings of LAZZARINI [1961b]. Attempts to stain myocytes for enzymes have not yet been made. The number of enzymes studied so far is small. Many more enzymes should be studied, and cytochemical reactions should be supplemented by chemical analyses of cells to facilitate comparisons with results obtained by studying whole arteries.

3. Amino Acids

The amino acid metabolism of nonvascular cells in culture has been studied extensively. Only limited work has been done with vascular cells. There is little data on amino acid turnover by vascular cells, and, for the most part, it is suggestive rather than conclusive.

POLLAK *et al.* [1960], ENGEL [1961], and ENGEL and POLLAK [1961a] used cells from one species, the rabbit, analyzed the nutrient but not the cells for free amino acids, and used mixed cultures but not pure cell lines. They did not apply quantitative methods. The nutrient was analyzed prior to inoculation, and 4, 8, and 12 days after the first outgrowth of cells. The explant was

---

Fig. 17. A. Two-dimensional electro-chromatograms of free amino acids in nutrient. Left, before inoculation with explant; right, after cell growth from rabbit aortic explant. *B* and *C.* Circular chromatograms of free amino acids in nutrient. *B.* Left part, before inoculation; right part, after cell growth from rabbit aortic plaque (darkest zone, cystathionine). *C.* Left part, after cell growth from intact rabbit aorta (darkest zone, glutathione); right part, after cell growth from rabbit aortic plaque (darkest zone, cystathionine).

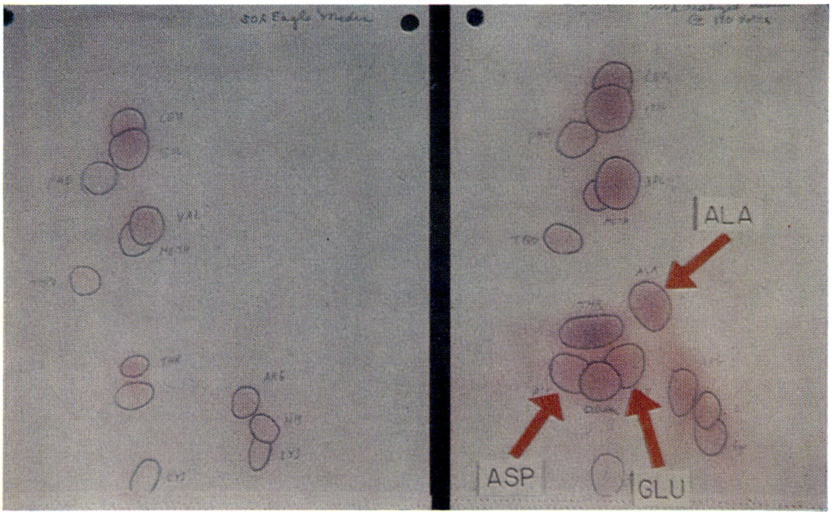

17 A

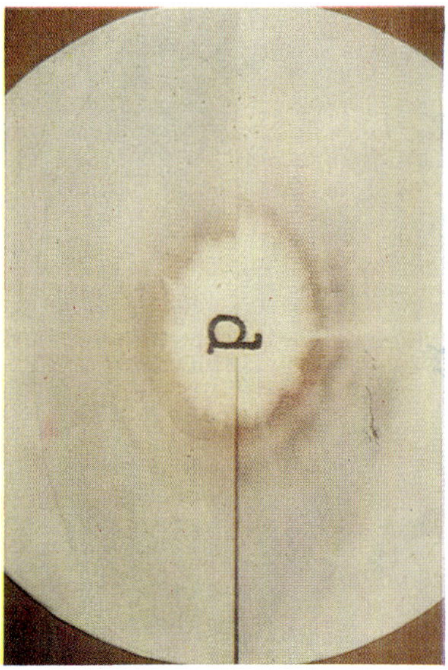

17 B

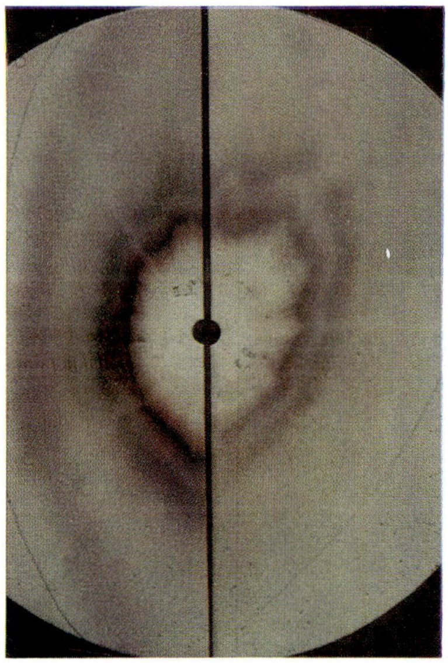

17 C

removed. Though the composition of the cell population changed in the 12-day period, smooth muscle cells were not present. Data on free amino acids in the nutrient (dessicated in a boiling water bath, with the residues suspended in 10% isopropanol) were obtained by a combination of paper electrophoresis and chromatography, and by high-speed centrifugal circular chromatography.

In spite of these limitations, the comparison of data on free amino acids in nutrient from cells originating from intact and altered aortae is interesting. There is a tendency toward numeric and qualitative increases in free amino acids following cell growth (fig. 17A). This increase is greater in cultures of cells from normal aortic sectors. Glutamic acid decreased and glutamine increased upon cell growth. (In this respect, rabbit aortic cells differ from nonvascular cells.) At the same time, α_2-globulin increased and β-globulin decreased progressively in the nutrient. The shifts paralleled the degree of cell proliferation.

ENGEL [1961] found that alanine was more prominent and threonine was more frequent in the media from altered explants. Aspartic acid decreased from the 1st to the 2nd change of the nutrient (day 4 and 8), probably because of utilization of this amino acid by the fibroblasts. Methionine, cystine, cysteine, glutamic acid, and glycine were often detected in the nutrient from the plaque cells. In contrast, valine was more often recovered in the nutrient from the control cells.

The observation was made by ENGEL [1961] that nutrient from cells grown from intact aortic sectors contained glutathione whereas that from cells grown from atherosclerotic sectors contained cystathionine (fig. 17B and C). It is interesting that those amino acids which comprise glutathione (α-glutamyl-cysteinyl-glycine)—especially, glycine—are found in the nutrient from cells of intact aortae less often than in the nutrient from plaque cells. This could indicate intracellular synthesis. Cystathionine (carboxyamino-propyl-S-cysteine) is a biosynthetic intermediate in methionine formation by mammalian cells. Its presence may indicate a metabolic block. Possibly, normal cells utilize methionine synthesized by different pathways: homoserin – thiomethylcysteine – methionine, or homoserin + S – homocysteine + CH_3 – methionine. Increased frequency of cystine and cysteine in the nutrient from plaque cells may be due to cystathionine cleavage: methionine or glucose – homocysteine + serine – cystathionine – homoserin + cystein – α-ketobutyric acid – α-aminobutyric acid.

WERTHESSEN [1961] suggested that S^{35} be added and also S^{35}-cysteine to shed light on the problem. The pathways from glutamine to glutamic acid

Glutathione and cystathionine pathways

Glutathione found in medium after growth of cells from intact aorta

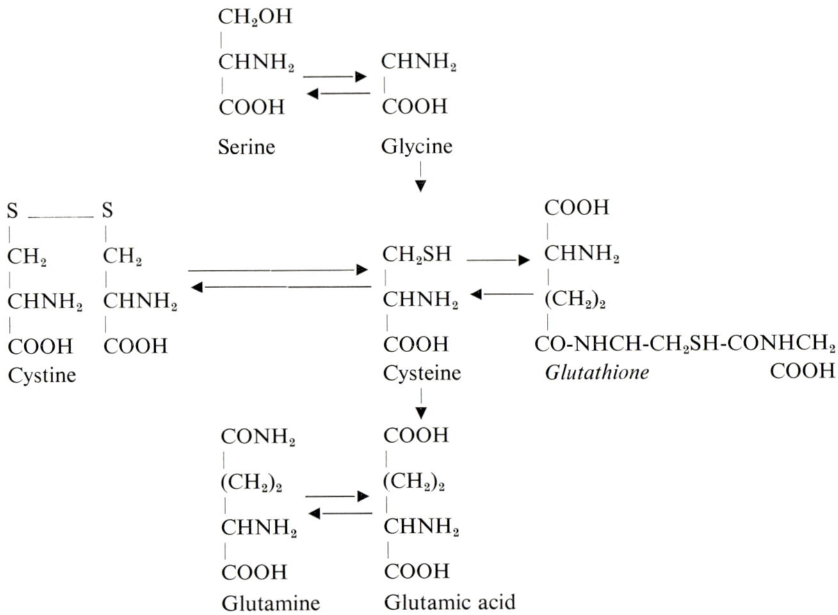

Cystathionine found in medium after growth of cells from altered aorta

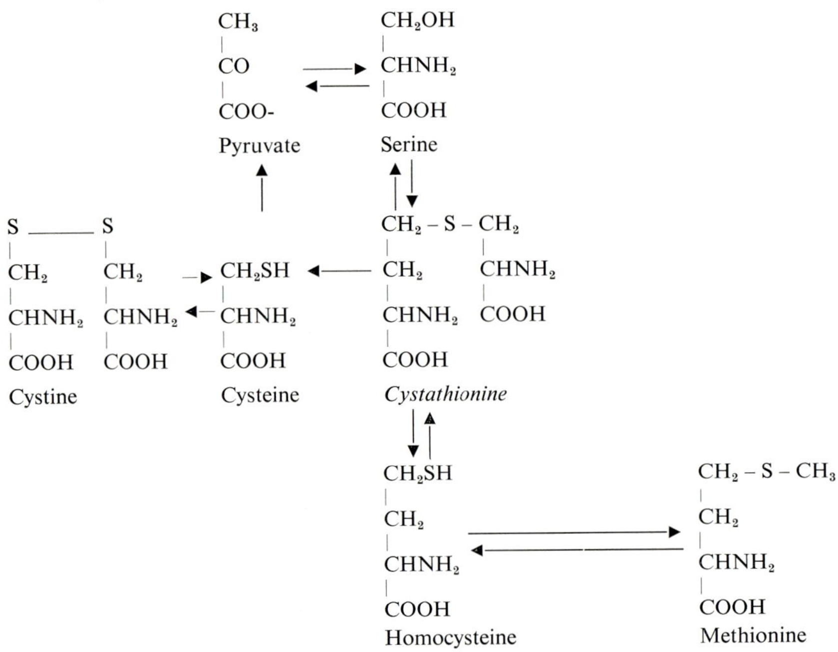

to acid mucopolysaccharides should be studied. Another profitable approach may be the *in vivo* administration of S^{35} and sulfur- or sulfhydril-containing amino acids to normal and hypercholesteremic rabbits—donors of explants for aortic cultures.

4. Lipoids

a) General Comments

In comparison with other facets of vascular cell metabolism, lipoids have been studied extensively. However, much remains to be done in this field. Generally, endothelial cells and fibroblasts have been used for studies. Smooth muscle cells have been studied only once. Fat-laden macrophages have not received special attention, although references to cells grown from atherosclerotic arteries imply the presence of such cells in cultures.

Many variations in the recorded observations of lipoids can be ascribed to methodology. Cells from several species have been used, but no attention has been paid to the age of the explant donors or to the calibre of the arteries used. No attention has been paid to the age of cells or cell populations, although this is an important factor in light of the spontaneous lipoid deposition in cells (fig. 14A). Cholesterol has been added in varying concentrations for varying lengths of time, in watery solutions and in alcoholic suspensions, singly or as lipoprotein, unlabeled and labeled in several ways. Hypercholesteremic serum and hyperlipemic serum have been added, prepared artificially, or as postprandial serum (after different diets). No attention has been paid to age or health of the subjects from whom blood was drawn for these experiments. Adsorption studies by HRŮZA *et al.* [1967] and lipfanogen studies by SIMMS [1936 and on] and LEWIS [1961] suggest that the donor's age and health are important factors in the adsorption and absorption of lipoids.

b) Incorporation of Unlabeled Lipoids

RUTSTEIN *et al.* [1958] observed intracellular lipoid deposits on the 4th to 5th day of incubation. Human aortic fibroblasts were exposed to alcoholic (0 mg, 1 mg, 2 mg, 3 mg, and 4 mg/100 ml nutrient) and aqueous (0 mg, 10 mg, 30 mg, 50 mg, and 70 mg) cholesterol suspensions. When, on the 8th day (series with alcoholic cholesterol) or on the 6th day (series with β-lipoprotein), the nutrient with 3 mg/100 ml (1st series) or 50 mg/100 ml (2nd series) was replaced by a cholesterol-free nutrient, incomplete reversal occurred within 5 days. However, no reduction of intracellular lipoid occurred when the original medium contained more than 3 mg of the alcoholic or more that 50 mg of the watery cholesterol suspension per 100 ml. Refeeding of cells with 50 mg of the watery suspension resulted in further lipoid deposition.

Similar clearing of cells was reported by LAZZARINI [1959], when he replaced the nutrient for human aortic cells, in which 0.1 ml of the medium had been substituted with 0.1 ml of watery cholesterol emulsion. Incubation of cells in cholesterol-free nutrient for 148 hours resulted in a reduction of intracellular lipoids. Temporary reduction was also obtained upon the addition of 0.1 ml of 5% dialyzed human serum albumin prior to the 120-hour incubation period in nutrient with cholesterol.

KOIDE and POLLAK [1963a] and KASAI *et al.* [1964] recorded the distribution of sudanophilic granules in endothelial cells, fibrocytes and macrophages grown from rabbit atherosclerotic aortae (fig. 18 A). They observed the distribution of lipoids in the 3 cell types under phase contrast illumination (fig. 19). In the macrophages, all lipoid was seen in the nucleus. In the endothelial cells, the luminescent material was in the nuclear membrane and the dense perinuclear zone of the cytoplasm. In the fibrocytes, it was in the juxtanuclear position, at both poles of the nucleus. There were differences in the amount and in the size of the fat droplets. The two methods of study, staining with Sudan Black B and phase contrast illumination, were supplementary to each other. In the evaluation of incorporation of lipoid and its removal, spontaneous lipoid deposition and artificial lipoid metamorphosis caused by additives to the nutrient must be considered.

c) Uptake of Radioactively Labeled Lipoids

Human and canine aortic endothelial cells and fibroblasts were exposed to radioactively labeled cholesterol at concentrations below 40 μg/ml by LAZZARINI [1961a, 1961c, 1961d, 1961e]. In 282 cultures, there was a strong uptake of the label by 7- to 10-day-old endothelial cells, but practically no uptake by fibroblasts. Uptake of lipoids occurred in two steps: First, phospholipoids and cholesterol present in the cell membrane were replaced by extracellular lipoids; next, lipoids passed into the cytoplasm at a gradient between the cell membrane and the subcellular fractions at 120 μg to 140 μg of the total lipoid concentration in 40 to 120 minutes.

Fig. 18. Distribution of sudanophilic matter in rabbit aortic cells. Culture, 6 days old. *A.* Endothelial cell (center), fibrocytes (left and bottom, part). *B.* Macrophage. Sudan black B (× 1260).

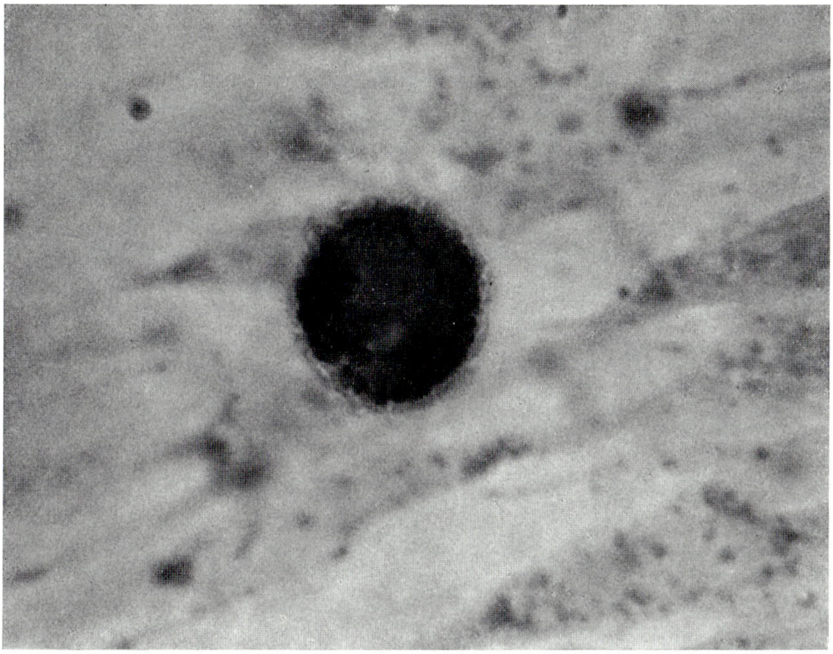

A

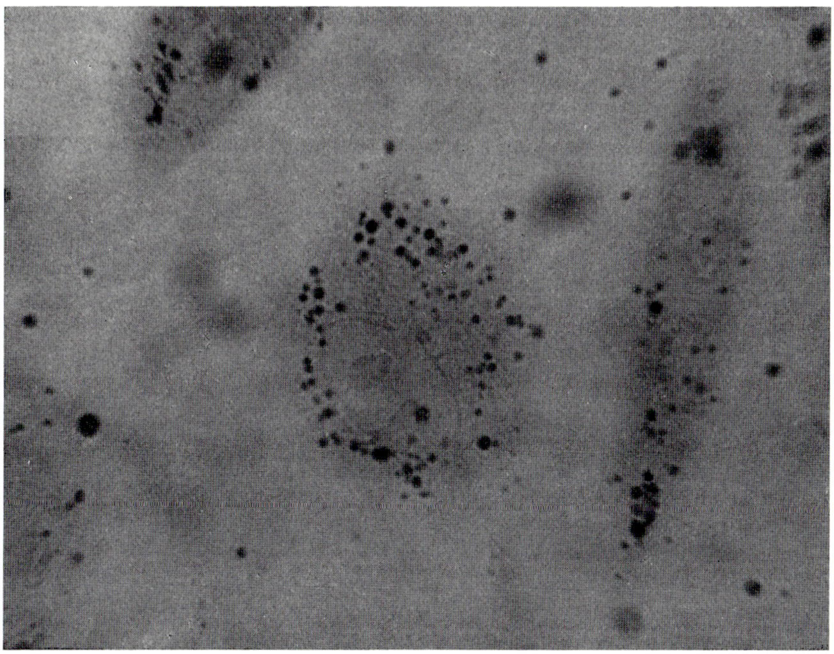

B

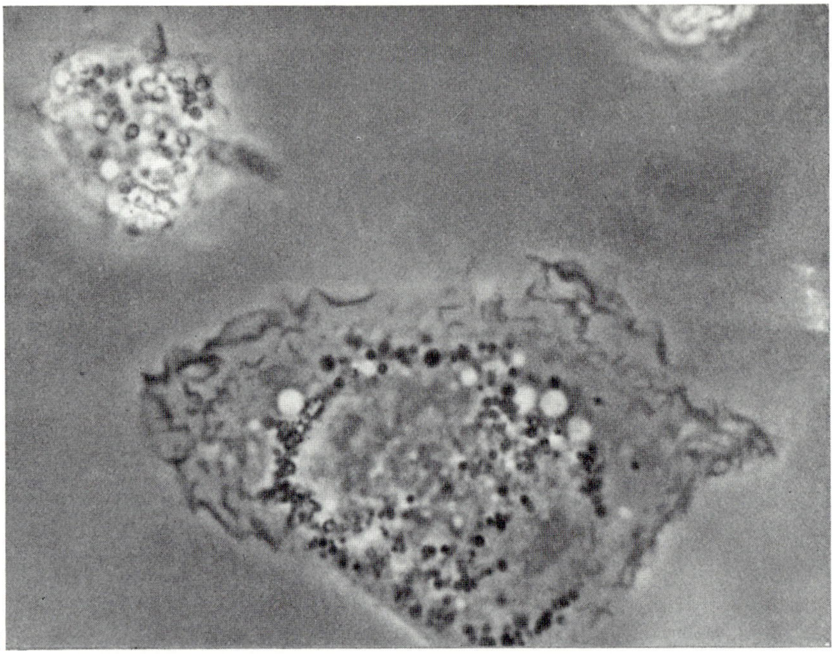

A

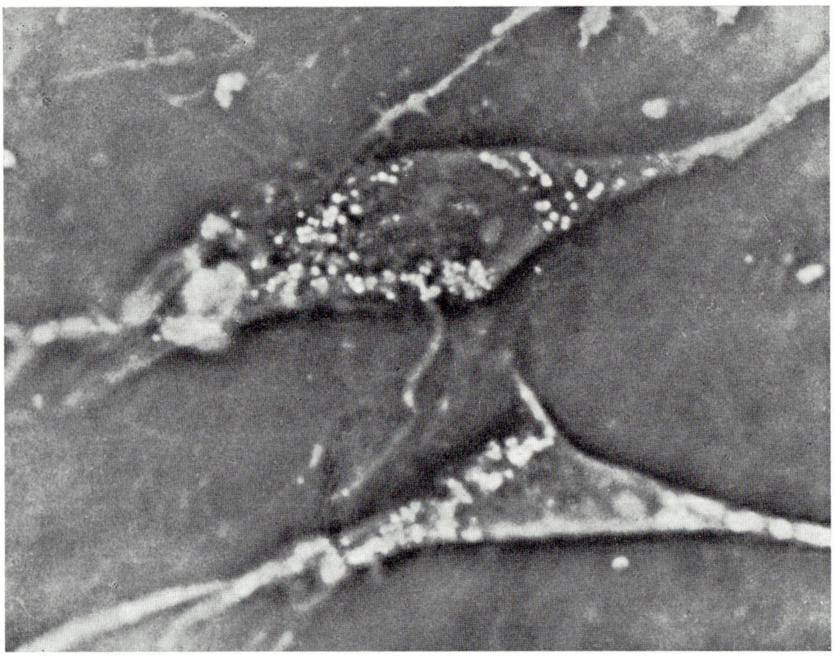

B

Upon incubation of cells in a mixture of ^{3}H-cholesterol and ^{131}I-serum protein, ROBERTSON [1965b, 1967] observed, by autoradiography and electronmicroscopy, that 'osmiphilic vacuoles' increased (this time) within 15 to 90 minutes. Simultaneously, microvilli appeared in 'atherophils'. Colloid carbon was used as the lipoprotein marker. After 30 minutes, the uptake of sterols was twice as high as the uptake of protein.

MURATA [1968] added C^{14}-acetate at 0.44 μc/ml and C^{14}-4-cholesterol at 0.1 μc/ml to chicken aortic endothelial cells. After 6 hours of incubation at 37° C, the uptake rate paralleled the incubation time.

d) Synthesis of Cellular Lipoids

Nutrient with 20^{5} cloned human aortic endothelial cells was used by LAZZARINI [1961a, 1962e, 1963c] for extensive studies of protein-bound cholesterol-7-α-H^{3} uptake and for intracellular cholesterol synthesis from sodium acetate-1-C^{14} and DL-mevalonic-2-C^{14}. He found that C^{14} incorporation decreased, while squalene H^{3} in the cells increased with increased oxygen tension. Conversely, as the oxygen concentration of the gas phase decreased, uptake of cholesterol increased. Reduction of DL-mevalonate-2-C^{14} and labeled CO_2 was proportional to the intracellular cholesterol concentration, which, in turn, was directly related to the length of incubation.

At an oxygen concentration below 10% the uptake of lipoid from α_2- or β-lipoprotein increased and the utilization of acetate decreased. At O_2 below 5%, acetate utilization decreased by 72.6 to 84.6%. At first, ROBERTSON [1965a, 1967] ascribed the intracellular increase of squalene (by 56.9 to 71.2%) to the modification of sterol biosynthesis by the hypoxia. Later [1968], he concluded that as O_2 decreased cell membrane permeability increased.

The concept of a balance between the availability of extracellular lipoids and intracellular lipoid synthesis was supported by a study with a single label by MURATA *et al.* [1966]. This team added human lipemic serum (total lipoid, 1080 mg/100 ml) to 5- to 7-day-old chicken aortic cells. Measured by C^{14}-acetate utilization, synthesis was accelerated on the 1st day, equilibrated in the 2nd day, and suppressed by 41% after 3 days of incubation—when the nutrient (MEM) contained 5% lipemic serum—and by 57%—

Fig. 19. Distribution of lipoid in rabbit aortic cells. Culture, 6 days old. *A.* Macrophage (upper left, round) and endothelial cell (large, polyhedric). *B.* Fibrocytes. Reverse phase contrast; stop-motion, cinephotomicrography (× 1260).

when it contained 10% lipemic serum. The suppression rates reflected the time elapsed between the incubation with lipemic serum and incubation with labeled acetate: The rates were 37% if the 2 incubations followed each other promptly, 30% if 1 day, 21% if 2 days, and 5–17% if 3 days had elapsed.

A dynamic balance, by a feed-back mechanism, between cholesterol storage and removal was postulated by LAZZARINI [1962b, 1963a] on the basis of observations that the incorporation of extracellular labeled lipoids inhibits lipoid synthesis [1962a]. ROBERTSON [1965a] spoke of homeostasis on the cellular level.

e) Transmembrane Movements of Lipoids

Intracellular accumulation of lipoids is regulated in several ways. It is dependent upon the availability of extracellular lipoids, the state of dispersion of the lipoids, and the length of time cells are exposed to those lipoids. The uptake increases with the degree of hypoxia and, concommitantly, intracellular synthesis decreases.

Using human and canine aortic explants, both normal and atherosclerotic, LAZZARINI [1960a, 1961a, 1961d, 1963c, 1963d] found that cations enhance the uptake of labeled lipoids whereas anions reduce it. After 18 hours incubation at pH 7.2, protamin sulfate 40 μg–80 μg/ml enhanced uptake by 21.4%, and esterified (methylated) bovine serum albumin 10 μg–30 μg/ml increased uptake by 32.7%; sodium stearate 25 μg–50 μg/ml reduced uptake by 51.9%, and N-acetylated bovine serum albumin 10 μg–50 μg/ml decreased uptake by 66.9%. Untreated amphoteric bovine serum albumin had no effect on lipoid uptake.

ROBERTSON [1965a, 1965b, 1967] determined that mucopolysaccharides of the ground substance inhibit lipoprotein entry into the arterial wall by regulating the transport of macromolecules. Earlier, LAZZARINI [1961b] had stated that the absorption of cholesterol from suspensions was paralleled by a reduction of oxidative processes and an increased production of MPS. The sequence of these events may be important to those who want to know whether the accumulation of arterial mucopolysaccharides precedes or follows the accumulation of lipoids.

f) Manipulation of Lipoid Movements

α) Heparin

The ability of heparin to clear hyperlipemic serum in the test tube has long been known. To test the influence of heparin on the loading and unloading of lipoid by vascular cells, LAZZARINI [1959] exposed human aortic endothelial cells to a mixture of 40 μg/ml cholesterol and 5 μg–10 μg/ml heparin. Such cells had fewer lipoid granules than cells exposed only to cholesterol. LAZZARINI [1961a, 1961b, 1962e, 1963b, 1963d] saw no effect when cholesterol was added first to the nutrient, and heparin was added 24 hours later, nor when heparin was added first and cholesterol later.

BRANWOOD [1961a, 1963] added 0.5 to 5 mg of heparin per 100 ml of nutrient, after feeding human aortic cells with hyperlipemic serum. He noted very rapid clearing of lipoid from the cells. FREEMAN *et al.* [1961] stated that heparin—a highly sulfated substance of high molecular weight, low osmotic pressure, and strong negative electric charge—does not enhance lipoid uptake by chicken aortic cells. HAUST [1961] questioned whether cysteine or cystine would have an effect similar to that of heparin. CURTIS and GALVIN [1963] exposed human and canine aortic fibroblasts to 3 mg cholesterol and 500 IU of heparin per 100 ml of nutrient, simultaneously. There was no effect on cholesterol deposit.

It appears that heparin can reduce uptake of cholesterol only when added to the nutrient simultaneously with cholesterol. LAZZARINI [1959] added cholesterol-7-α-^{3}H and heparin (10 mg/ml); there was no significant uptake of the label after 170 minutes. On addition of cholesterol-4-C^{14} and heparin, uptake was insignificant after 180 minutes. From mixtures of 40 μg labeled serum lipoprotein and 50 μg heparin, uptake was 36.2% lower after 12 hours and 71.1% lower after 22 hours than in cultures without heparin. At first, LAZZARINI [1959] thought that doses over 10 mg were toxic; later [1961b, 1963c] he found that heparin had no toxic effect on vascular cells.

β) Mucopolysaccharides

The characteristics of heparin led to the study of mucopolysaccharides. LAZZARINI [1961b] stated that under the influence of heparin metachromatic granules appear on the cell membrane of endothelial cells. KOIDE and POLLAK [1963] found MPS in the perinuclear zone of most normal rabbit aortic endothelial cells and in all fat-laden macrophages, but not in fibrocytes. KASAI *et al.* [1964] found that the nuclear membrane of endothelial cells gave positive reactions with Toluidine Blue and with the periodic acid-Schiff stain.

FREEMAN *et al.* [1961] used extracts of calf aortae—rich in MPS—and noted a clearing effect on lipoid-laden chicken aortic cells. MORRISON *et al.* [1963] loaded 5- to 6-day-old chicken aortic cells with human lipemic serum, and then incubated the cells for 72 hours with 4 extracts of dried calf aortae, with condroitin sulfate A (CS-A) and B (CS-B), and with IN-379 (pimentine HCl). Total lipoids decreased from 100 mg to 82 mg/100 ml upon treatment with aortic extract No. 1 and CS-A. CS-B had no effect, and IN-379 enhanced lipoid deposits. MURATA *et al.* [1966] noted that on addition of CS-A to chicken aortic cells lipoid synthesis increased by 10%–20%, and by 7%–10% upon addition of CS-C. Increases in lipoid synthesis by these substances is in accord with reduction of lipoid incorporation by the same substances.

γ) Histamine

Histamine, 0.1 μg/ml, reduced by 40% the synthesis of neutral fat, phospholipoids, and free sterols in 2 generations of chicken aortic cells incubated for 3 days by MURATA *et al.* [1966]. This effect could be correlated with 2 factors: The histamine concentration and the incubation period. MURATA *et al.* [1967a] first added 0.1 μg histamine/ml MEM with 5% calf serum and incubated for 3 days/37° C; they then replaced the medium with a nutrient containing 0.44 μc/ml of Na-acetate-C^{14} and incubated for 6 h/37° C. The histamine effect could be neutralized by diphenylhydramine HCl (DPH), an antihistamine. After 2 days of incubation with histamine, the synthesis of lipoids was 65%, compared with 100% of controls, and after additional 2-day incubation with DPH.

δ) Hormones

Clinical and experimental experiences with various steroid hormones prompted a number of investigators to test the effect of hormones on the lipoid metabolism of arterial cells in culture. LAZZARINI [1959, 1961d, 1963] found that α-estradiol prevents the uptake of lipoids by human aortic endothelial cells on the microsomal level, and that progesterone is low in inducing clearing. LAZZARINI [1961a, 1963] determined that 0.4 μg/ml is the effective clearing dose of estradiol benzoate. BRANWOOD [1961a, 1963] used 0.05 mg/100 ml nutrient and observed clearing of endothelial cells in 48 hours. Simultaneous use of the hormone and human lipemic serum blocked lipoid deposits. CURTIS and GALVIN [1963], upon the simultaneous addition of 3 mg cholesterol and 0.1 mg testosterone propionate, serum gonadotropin, stilbestrol, or prednisone, saw no effect on lipoid uptake by human and canine aortic fibroblasts. They observed some effect when hexosterol was added, and very good results with progesterone and methyl-testosterone. ACTH corticotropin (0.15 IU) and L-thyroxin (3 μg) had no effect. Insulin (0.2 IU) addition was fairly effective, with 1+ lipoid deposit (on a scale of – to 4+).

Adrenalin and noradrenalin did not affect lipoid synthesis from C^{14}-acetate by chicken aortic cells, according to MURATA *et al.* [1966]. Cortisone augmented the uptake of labeled lipoproteins by human aortic cells, according to LAZZARINI [1961d]. CURTIS and GALVIN [1963] found that 0.1 mg cortisone plus 0.3 mg cholesterol caused marked (3+) lipoid deposit in aortic fibroblasts. The enhancement of intracellular lipoid accumulation by a mixture of human lipemic serum and 10 μg to 50 μg of cortisone was ascribed by BRANWOOD [1963] to the toxic effect of cortisone on human aortic endothelial cells.

ε) Adenosinephosphates

On the assumption that adenosinetriphosphate (ATP) regulates the splitting of lipoproteins, ROBERTSON [1965b, 1967] added 10 μg to 40 μg of ATP/ml nutrient. C^{14}-cholesterol uptake was accelerated within 30 minutes. (The effect can be blocked by AT-phosphatase.)

The concept of cellular homeostasis—a balance between cholesterol uptake and synthesis—advanced by LAZZARINI [1965a and on] seems plausible. However, the reports by MURATA *et al.* [1966, 1967] that 10 μg to 20 μg ATP/ml nutrient significantly increased the synthesis from acetate-^{14}C of neutral fat, phospholipoids, and free sterols by chicken aortic cells seems to be in direct conflict. Reconciliation could be achieved by uniform experiments: ROBERTSON [1965b, 1967] incubated for 30 minutes; MURATA *et al.* [1966, 1967] for 6 hours. ATP had no effect on lipoid synthesis after 2 hours but was effective after 4 and 6 hours' incubation. ADP and AMP were about half as effective as ATP. CURTIS and GALVIN [1963] recorded ++ fat deposit (and 4+ necrosis) of human and dog aortic fibroblasts upon addition of 3 mg cholesterol and 10 mg ATP/100 ml nutrient.

η) Serotonin, Puromycin

Acceleration of lipoid synthesis (30 to 35%), by chicken aortic cells in F^1 and F^2 was noted by MURATA *et al.* [1966] upon the addition of 10 μg of serotonin (5-hydroxy-tryptamine)/ml nutrient.

Puromycin, a cellular poison and an enzyme inhibitor, was added by MURATA *et al.* [1967] to cultures of chicken aortic cells. They found that 50 μg/ml of puromycin depressed sterol synthesis from I-^{14}C-acetate (0.44 μc/ml) by 47% in 2 hours, and total lipoid synthesis by 18% in 3 hours, compared to controls. ROBERTSON [1968] stated that puromycin (and also aureomycin) inhibits the formation of 'foam cells' from endothelial cells, blocking, apparently, the uptake of extracellular cholesterol. It seems unlikely that the same compound (puromycin) depresses both uptake [MURATA, 1967] and synthesis [ROBERTSON, 1968]. It must be noted that conflicting results are based on experiments which differ as to the origin of cells, dosage, and incubation time.

L. Fatty Acids, Diets

1. Unsaturated and Saturated Fatty Acids

Long before nutritionists suggested that animal fats, containing saturated fatty acids, promote the absorption of cholesterol (and subsequently enhance atherogenesis), and that vegetable fats with unsaturated fatty acids have the opposite effect, pertinent experiments with aortic cell cultures had been made. SIMMS [1937] observed that human serum containing salts of fatty acids resulted in greater deposition of lipoids in chicken aortic fibroblasts. SIMMS *et al.* [1947] found that of the unsaturated fatty acids, Na oleate was the most potent lipoid depositing agent, whereas the acids from linseed oil produced little uptake of lipoids, and Na hendeconate had no lipfanogenic effect. Of the saturated acids, Na stearate caused more deposit than palmitate, myristate and laureate. SIMMS [1961] reported that the serum of rats which had been fed animal fats contained 43% more lipfanogens and 55% less antilipfanogen than serum of rats fed vegetable fats.

BRANWOOD [1961a, 1963] treated human aortic cells with 0.1 ml of human lipemic serum. One serum pool contained 1600 mg lipoids/100 ml (after ingestion of 85 g animal fat), another serum contained 800 mg lipoids/100 ml (after ingestion of corn oil with 80% linoleic acid). The first serum induced lipoid granules in endothelial cells (but not in fibroblasts); the second serum had no effect on lipoid deposits.

Beta-lipoprotein (10 mg–70 mg/100 ml) was added to cultures with human aortic fibroblasts, by RUTSTEIN *et al.* [1958]. The more lipoid was added the greater the uptake by cells. The simultaneous addition of 1 mg linoleic acid prevented cellular lipoidosis almost completely. Mixtures of 3 mg cholesterol and 1 mg stearic acid/100 ml resulted in potentiation of deposits; mixtures of 3 mg cholesterol and 1 mg linoleic acid completely inhibited deposits. The minimum dose of linoleic acid to influence cholesterol deposits was 5 mg/100 ml.

LAZZARINI [1959, 1961a, 1961b] tested the influence of fatty acids on cholesterol uptake by human aortic cells. Using 40 μg of cholesterol plus 1 μg to 10 μg linoleic acid/ml nutrient, he found diminished uptake. Increased uptake resulted from 40 μg of cholesterol plus 1 μg to 5 μg of palmitic or butyric acid. The fatty acids had no effect if added 24 hours after the addition of cholesterol to nutrient. BRANWOOD [1961a, 1963] observed the clearing of human endothelial cells within 48 hours with 25 mg or as little as 1 mg of arachidonic acid/100 ml. Phospholipoids, containing varying amounts of arachidonic acid, had a clearing effect comparable to that of pure arachidonic acid.

Human and canine aortic fibroblasts were used by CURTIS and GALVIN [1963] to evaluate a large number of chemicals, including 10 fatty acids. Phospholipoid-linoleic acid (1.5 mg) was most effective with regard to inhibition of lipoid deposits. Pure linoleic acid (1 mg), stearic acid (1 mg) as octadeca-trans-13-ene 9,11-diyonic acid, and palmitic acid (1 mg) as hexadeca-cis-2, cis-4 were also effective when added together with 3 mg cholesterol. Maize oil with linoleic esters and mono- and diglycerides of linoleic acid had no effect.

2. Postprandial Serum

Human postprandial serum was added by SIMMS [1937] to chicken aortic fibroblasts and by BRANWOOD [1961a, 1963] to human aortic endothelial cells. Varions fatty acids and cholesterol suspensions were tested by SIMMS *et al.* [1947, 1954] on chicken fibroblasts, mixtures by RUTSTEIN *et al.* [1958] on human fibroblasts, and by LAZZARINI [1959, 1961a, 1961b] on human aortic endothelial cells. All results pointed to lipoid deposition by saturated fatty acids and a lesser deposition by polyunsaturated fatty acids.

In a sophisticated study, RUTSTEIN *et al.* [1964] tested the blood of 15 men, 30 to 60 years old. The group included 2 men with diabetes mellitus and 1 with myocardial infarction. Thirty-five sera, after fat or carbohydrate meals, or after prolonged fasting, were obtained several times over a 24-hour period. The sera were used as a replacement for 40% (volume) of nutrients with human and with Rhesus aortic fibroblasts. A base line was obtained from the results with fasting serum, although there was considerable variation in the individual responses.

RUTSTEIN *et al.* [1964] observed maximum lipoid deposits upon the addition of serum of men who consumed a 2000 caloric diet of polyunsaturated fatty acids. (It compared with results upon exposure of cells to cholesterol suspension.) Heavy lipoid deposits followed the addition of serum after ingestion of 2000 calories of butter or 1000 calories of safflower oil. Serum after 1000 to 2000 caloric coconut oil meals caused less deposit. Usually, maximum deposits occurred on the addition of serum taken 6 hours after the meal. In all series, the base line was reached by serum obtained 24 hours after the meal. Serum obtained after prolonged fasting caused an increase in lipoid deposits. A 2000 caloric carbohydrate meal reduced lipoid deposits below the base level, abruptly for the first 3 hours, then slowly for 6 hours, with a slight rise between the 6th and the 9th hour.

Lipoid deposits correlated best with blood triglyceride levels, according to Rutstein *et al.* [1964]. Yet, prolonged fasting and 2000 caloric carbohydrate meals yielded sera which enhanced lipoid deposits, although blood triglycerides were stable. Cellular lipoidosis correlated also fairly well with blood total lipoids, less with phospholipoids, and not at all with cholesterol.

Another study was performed with serum samples of 1 man. At 9 hours, postprandial lipoid deposits were lower on addition of serum after a 2000 caloric carbohydrate meal than on addition of serum after a 1000 caloric carbohydrate meal. The deposit-reducing effect of the two serum samples equalized if blood was taken 12 hours after the meals. Rutstein *et al.* [1967] also used the serum of 5 diabetic men. After insulin administration, the serum of these men acted in the same manner as serum of nondiabetic men; without insulin, results of the serum samples on lipoid deposits in culture cells were erratic.

Rutstein *et al.* [1964] developed a hypothesis that on prolonged fasting, body cells are deprived of a dietary source of energy and compensate by storing lipoids. After a carbohydrate meal, alimentary hyperglycemia suppresses the release of fats from storage and therefore cells have to utilize carbohydrates instead. One must ask why this reaction should be peculiar to arterial cells and to human embryonic muscle cells which were, according to Rutstein *et al.* [1964] the only cells among 13 human cell lines reacting in this manner.

An explanation was also sought for the paradoxical effect of serum after ingestion of polyunsaturated fatty acids, namely its enhancing of lipoid deposits. On the basis of long-term studies, epidemiologists suggested a beneficial effect of polyunsaturated fatty acids. In contrast, the cited experiments with tissue culture cells are short-term studies of 3 daily fat tides. Indirect support for the concept of fat tides was provided by Castelli *et al.* [1966]. After fasting, serum nonesterified fatty acids (NEFA) varied from person to person, between 554 mEq and 988 mEq (average, 679 mEq), and the inter-subject range was 602 mEq to 1068 mEq (average, 774 mEq). After a sunflower oil diet, NEFA always increased, with a 9-hour peak. Following a carbohydrate meal, NEFA decreased in 10 out of 11 subjects. Prolonged fasting caused increases in all 11. The parallel between serum NEFA and cellular lipoid deposits was evident.

No matter how plausible the experimental results with postprandial serum may be and how convincing the explanation of the results of RUTSTEIN *et al.* [1964, 1967], the fact remains that they are at variance with the reports of others who have added various sera to vascular cell cultures. These results also differ from earlier findings by the same research team and by others who have tried fatty acids as additives to arterial cells. Only one set of results can be correct. To arrive at a final decision, it is necessary to repeat these studies with postprandial serum and fatty acids, using radioactively labeled compounds. Endothelial cells and smooth muscle cells should be used, instead of arterial fibroblasts, for future investigations.

M. Cytopharmacology

All the attempts to delay or inhibit the incorporation of nonlabeled lipoids, to block the uptake of radioactively labeled lipoids, and to suppress lipoid synthesis by vascular cells, could be included under the heading of cytopharmacology.

It is unfortunate that CURTIS and GALVIN [1963], who tested 125 inorganic and organic chemicals and biologicals, used fibroblasts as their test cells, since this is the least suited cell type for the study of lipoids. In their experiments, aortic cells of men and dogs reacted alike. Three-week-old cultures were divided into 4 series: one, with 1% alcohol, one, with 3 mg cholesterol/100 ml of nutrient, one, with a test substance, -in 1/300 of the clinical dosage-, and one with 3 mg cholesterol and the test substance. Cellular lipoids and cell necrosis were rated on a scale up to 4+.

Some of the results obtained by CURTIS and GALVIN [1963], namely those with fatty acids, hormones, ATP, and heparin, have been included in a previous chapter (cf. chapter K, f). Several compounds which have been considered useful in clinical trials gave good results in cultures, especially linoleic acid (1 mg) and 'essential' linoleic phospholipoids (1.5 mg). Pyridoxine.HCl (0.2 IU), trypsin (1 mg), cholic acid (1 mg), potassium chloride (6.3 mg), magnesium sulfate (33 mg), and penicillin (4000 IU) also reduced lipoid deposits when added to nutrient simultaneously with 3 mg of cholesterol/100 ml.

Inorganic salts, other than KCl and Mg_2SO_4, had only a slight effect. Antibiotics, other than penicillin, enhanced lipoid deposits. Some of the compounds which have often been used in clinical studies gave disappointing results in *in vitro* experiments. Triparanol (in 3 doses, 0.5 mg, 1 mg, and 5 mg) caused maximum lipoid deposits and necrosis. Upon the addition of methionine (20 mg) or heparin (500 IU) intracellular lipoid was rated as 3+, α-tocopherol (2 mg), as 4+.

The second pertinent reference was made by ROBERTSON [1968a]. Ethyl-α-p-chlorophenoxyisobutyrate (CPIB) and 7-α-^{3}H-cholesterol (40 mc/ml) were added to human aortic 'intimacytes'. Significant inhibition of sterol uptake was noted if incubation with CPIB preceded the addition of labeled cholesterol. Partial inhibition took place if CPIB and cholesterol were added together to the nutrient. No inhibition was noted on autoradiographic examination of the cells if CPIB addition followed the incubation with cholesterol.

Vascular cytopharmacology has not been exhausted as a research tool.

N. Cytotoxicology

Some of the compounds which were used in the attempts to influence the transport of lipoids have a more or less pronounced toxic effect on vascular cells *in vitro*. The reaction of arterial cells to cytotoxins is not very different from the reactions of other cells. However, the sensitivities of the 4 types of cells grown from arteries differ quantitatively. Some compounds are mitotic poisons, some a growth inhibitor, some are nuclear poisons, cytoplasmic poisons, and enzymatic poisons. The ultimate effect of cytotoxins is cytolysis.

1. Cobalt Salts

A mucopolysaccharide-producing strain of human aortic fibroblasts was subjected by LAZZARINI and WEISSMANN [1960] to polyvalent cobalt salts. HeLa cells, which do not secrete MPS, were used as controls. Trivalent hexammoniacobalt chloride, $Co(NH_3)_6Cl_3$, induced, in a dose of 5 μg/ml for 13 hours at 37°C, large cytoplasmic vacuoles with metachromatic granules, but no nuclear changes. Hexavalent hexol nitrate, $[CO(OH)_6.(Co\ en_2)_3](NO_3)_6$, in a 5 μg dose, induced intranuclear granules, but no cytoplasmic damage; in a 50 μg/ml dose, large bubbles appeared in the cell membrane, but the cytoplasm was not affected. Alterations persisted for 120 hours. At 100 μg/ml, the trivalent salt inhibited growth; the hexavalent salt did not inhibit growth of aortic cells (HeLa cells underwent cytolysis.) $CaCl_2$,

260 μg/ml, inhibited growth but did not cause morphologic changes; nickelous ammonium bromide, 200 μg/ml, caused a similar effect.

2. Nicotine, Cigarette Smoke Condensate

The implication of cigarette smoking in atherogenesis prompted studies with nicotine, and with cigarette smoke condensate. Mixed populations—without smooth muscle cells—from intact and atherosclerotic explants of rabbit aortae were studied. POLLAK [1961], POLLAK and KOKUBU [1961], and KOKUBU and POLLAK [1962] added 0.04 ml of nicotine solutions (1:40,000, 1:10,000, 1:5,000, 1:2,500 and 1:1,000) to 100 ml of nutrient. The amounts of nicotine added were 1,400 μg, 560 μg, 280 μg, 140 μg, and 35 μg, respectively. If nicotine was added to nutrient before planting, there was, above concentrations of 1:2,500, marked reduction in the number of successful cultures and cell growth retardation. The higher the nicotine concentration, the shorter the life span of cells and the more severe the morphologic damage. If nicotine was added on the 4th day after planting, growth curves were depressed and morphologic alterations were prominent. Addition of 1:5000 or 1:2500 solutions of nicotine on the 7th day after inoculation of the medium caused only degeneration of endothelial cells.

In all experiments, endothelial cells were more sensitive than fibroblasts. Cells which appeared morphologically intact were affected metabolically—as demonstrated by consistent increases in glutamic acid in the nutrient—in comparison to the controls. Aortic and myocardial cells from hypercholesteremic rabbits were more sensitive to nicotine than cells from normocholesteremic rabbits. Their vulnerability must be ascribed to 'sensitization' by hypercholesteremia.

This concept found support by the disclosure of ADACHI *et al.* [1966] that the addition of nicotine depressed the respiration of tissues (aorta, heart, cornea, trachea, and liver) from hypercholesteremic animals significantly more than that of analogous tissues from control rabbits. The respiration quotients of aortic tissues were 26% that of liver tissues of normo- and mildly hypercholesteremic rabbits, and 20% in severly hypercholesteremic rabbits. This ratio remained fairly constant upon addition of nicotine solutions of various strength. Comparison with a study of the metabolism of nicotine by tissue slices from 8 sites of 3 species made by MILLER and LARSON [1953] is of interest. Interspecies and interorgan differences were observed. In all species, the liver metabolized nicotine more rapidly than

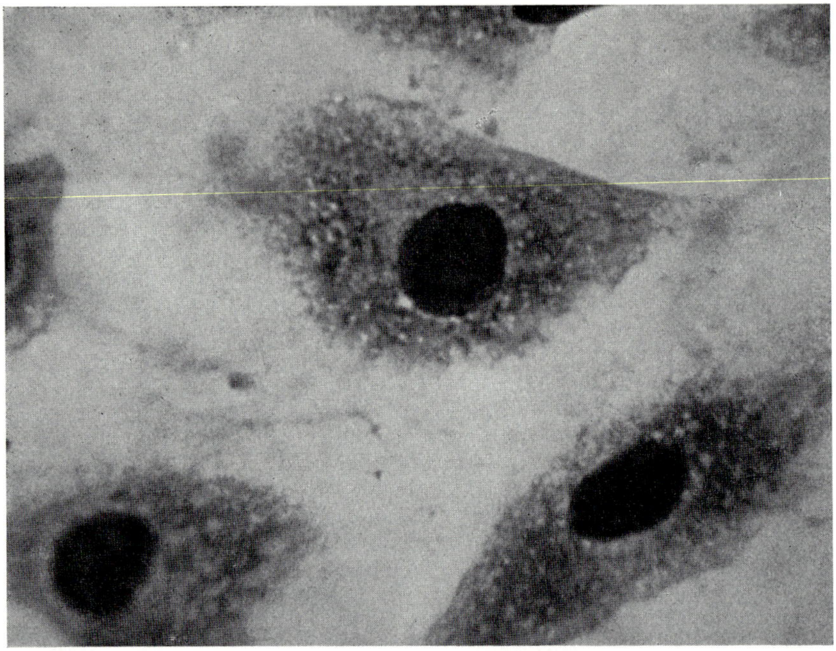

A

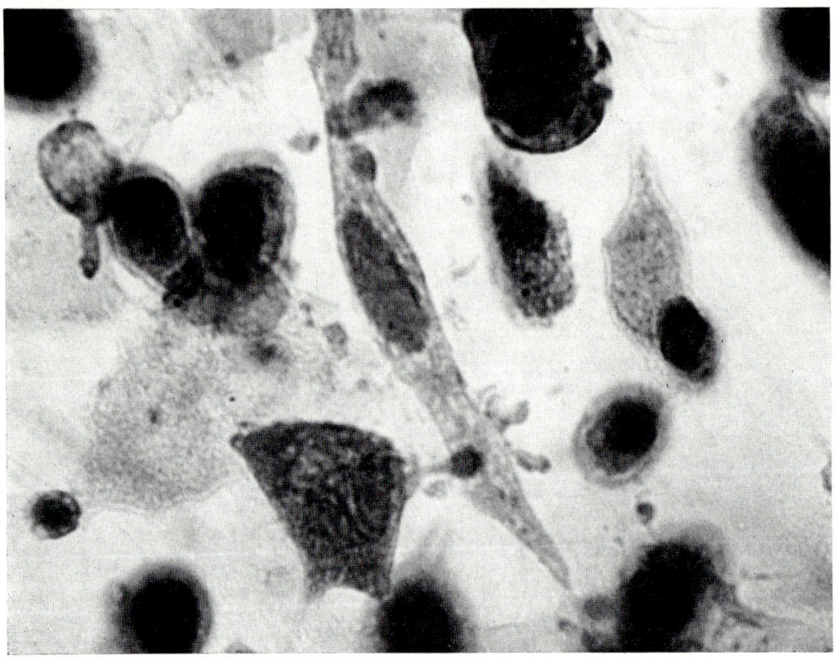

B

other tissues. The amounts of nicotine detoxified by 1 g of tissue in 3 h/37° C averaged for dog, rabbit and cat livers, 505 μg, 504 μg and 323 μg, for dog, rabbit and cat aortae, 217 μg, 164 μg, and 123 μg. Aortic slices metabolized 31, 32 and 35% less nicotine than liver slices.

Cytoplasmic alterations were, at first, an increase in number and size of granules, next, an increase in the size of vacuoles with expansion of vacuoles from the perinuclear zone toward the cell membrane. This was accompanied by pyknosis and karyorrhexis. Upon degranulation, lipoid particles appeared in the nutrient. 'Giant' cells with several huge vacuoles formed just prior to cytolysis (fig. 22A). The motility of cells diminished rapidly as the cells underwent explosive cytolysis on contact with nicotine solution, as shown by POLLAK and BURNS [1965] (fig. 22B).

On removal of the nicotine solution and replacement of the medium by fresh nutrient, the cells recovered (unless damage had progressed to vacuolization and pyknosis). The recovery of endothelial cells was poor in comparison with fibroblasts. Upon recovery, proliferation resumed. The effects of nicotine correlated with dosage and length of exposure; recovery rates correlated inversely with dosage and time.

Composite cigarette smoke condensate (CSC) from 4 types of cigarettes was tested by KOKUBU *et al.* [1961], and by KOIDE and POLLAK [1963]. The strength of the CSC was adjusted to the strength of nicotine. The range was 4.76 λ to 0.075 λ (equal to 7.4 μg to 1.1 μg/ml nicotine). CSC was added to the nutrient before planting, and every 3 to 4 days thereafter. Parallel to the increased doses, there was a decrease in the number of successful cultures and a retardation of cell growth. Cells from hypercholesteremic rabbits (850 mg/100 ml) were inhibited more than cells from normocholesteremic (55 mg/100 ml) rabbits. When CSC (2.4 λ) was added on the 7th day after planting, morphologic changes were, within 1 hour, similar to those induced by nicotine. On single exposure to 2.4 λ, for 3 hours, on the 7th day, proliferation was not disrupted, but structural alterations were observed. Recovery of cells occurred, lest damage had progressed to vacuolization and pyknosis.

Fig. 20. A. Rabbit aortic endothelial cells exposed to CS/100 for 24 hours. Culture, 5 days old. Giemsa stain (×500). *B.* Rabbit aortic endothelial cells (shrinking) and a myocyte (budding) exposed to CS/100 for 24 hours. Culture, 14 days old. Pollak's trichrome stain (×400). [Enlarged figures 5 and 6 in KASAI, T. and POLLAK, O.J., 1964; reproduced with permission of the publishers of the Tohoku med. J.]

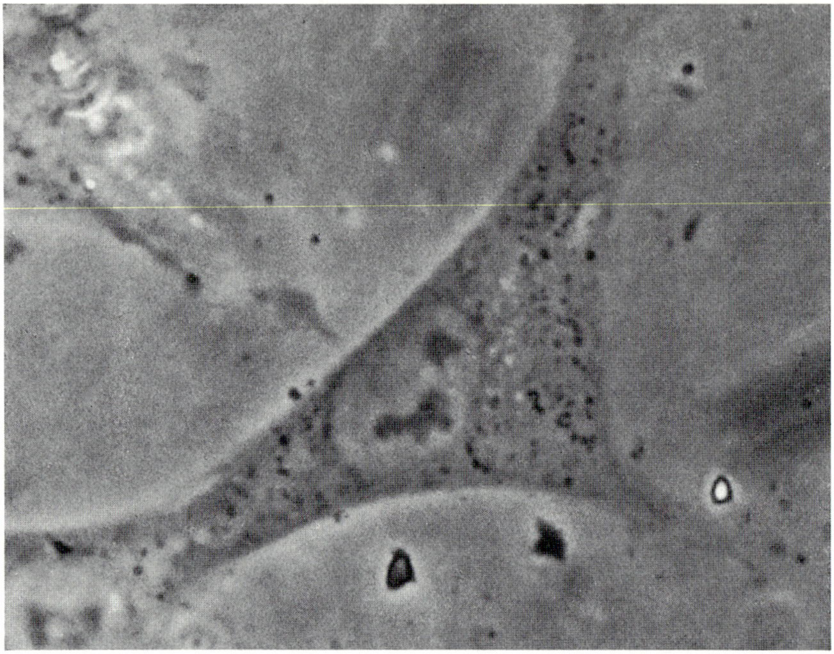

A

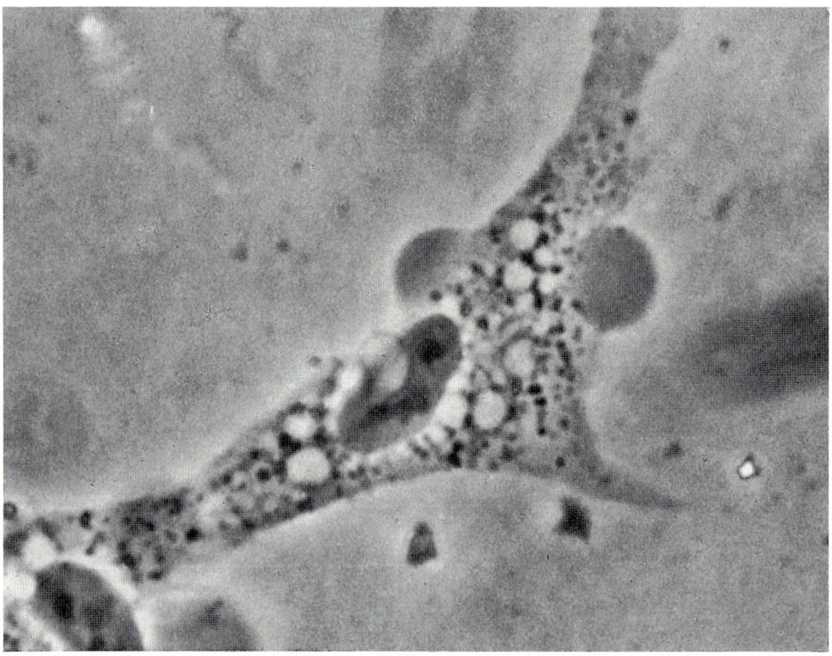

B

KOIDE and POLLAK [1963] compared the effect of CSC from 4 types of cigarettes—regular (R), denicotinized (DN), filter-tipped (FT), and denicotinized and filter-tipped (DN-FT). The growth curves were comparable, regardless of the source of CSC. Morphologic damage was far greater if CSC from untipped cigarettes was used. Denicotinization had no beneficial effect. Recovery of cells was incomplete after exposure to CSC from untipped cigarettes. CSC from tipped cigarettes 'paralyzed' the cells, and proliferation was temporarily arrested; within 3 days, the growth curves resembled those of the control cultures. CSC was 30 times more toxic than nicotine. This was ascribed to the particulate matter in the condensate.

KASAI and POLLAK [1964] used a home-made apparatus to produce cigarette smoke (CS) from denicotinized cigarettes. Smoke from 1 cigarette was added to 10 ml of nutrient, and the pH adjusted to 7.4. By dilution with fresh nutrient, CS/50 to CS/400 were obtained, and these solutions contained 15 μg to 1.875 μg of nicotine. CS introduced before inoculation and 3 to 4 days later resulted in growth inhibition at CS/50, in growth depression at CS/100 and CS/200, and in normal growth at CS/400. Addition of CS on the 7th day after planting stopped all growth at CS/50. At CS/100, growth curves dropped sharply to 0; at CS/200, curves flattened, while at CS/400, growth curves matched those of controls. A single dose of CS/100 was applied to a 7-day-old culture for 72, 24, and 3 hours. Only the 3-hour exposure did not leave permanent damage.

On exposure to CSC, endothelial cells first expanded, then shrank. Their cell membrane thickened. Young cells were damaged less than older cells and recovered easier (fig. 20A). Smooth muscle cells lost myofilaments, shrank, and developed cytoplasmic protrusions. Comparing the effects of nicotine, CSC, and CS, KOKUBU *et al.* [1961] noted that the budding effect was only seen on exposure to CS (fig. 20B). The nuclear membrane of fibrocytes thickened within 30 minutes, budding and vacuolization began within 60 minutes, and cell contraction and pyknosis developed in 160 minutes on contact with CSC (fig. 21). Damage by cigarette smoke exceeded that caused by cigarette smoke condensate, but not by the magnitude by which the condensate differed from nicotine.

Fig. 21. Rabbit aortic fibroblasts. *A.* Before exposure to CS/100 (7.5 μg nicotine). *B.* 70 minutes after exposure to CS/100 (7.5 μg nicotine) for 24 hours. Culture, 13 to 14 days old. Unstained (×1200). Time-lapse cinephotomicrography. [Enlarged from figures 7A and 7C in KASAI, T. and POLLAK, O.J., 1964; reproduced with permission of the publishers of the Tohoku J. exp. Med.]

Table IX. Aortic fatty acids of 2 pigeon breeds

Fatty acids	(% of total)	Homogenates WC[1]	Homogenates SR[2]	Fibroblasts WC[1]	Fibroblasts SR[2]
Stearic	C 18:1	24.0	19.6	30.3	29.2
Oleic	C 18:2	22.7	30.0	22.3	21.9
Arachidonic	C 20:4	8.7	8.5	0	7.7

[1] WC = White Carneau — [2] SR = Show Racer

O. Cytogenetics

Two references to the chromosomes of aortic cells *in vitro* were made. Robertson [1965a] did not find chromosomal aberrations in cloned cells studied from 10 weeks to 29 months. Priest and Priest [1964] counted 42 chromosomes in F^1 through F^{15} of rat aortic fibroblasts during 4 months of observation. A search for chromosomal differences should be made by comparing cells from related species which differ as to the incidence of atherosclerosis.

An example of such differences are the susceptible White Carneau (WC) and the resistant Show Racer (SR) pigeons. Smith *et al.* [1965] compared the results of fatty acid assays in homogenates of aortae of the 2 breeds with the results of fatty acid assays of fibroblasts cultured from aortae of the 2 breeds (table IX, very much condensed from the original report).

The absence of arachidonic acid in cells from the susceptible breed may be significant. Seegers [1961] stated that enzymatic activity is genetically determined and regulated by hormones. Arachidonic acid is a part of the phospholipoids of the cell membrane and of the mitochondria, with the latter playing a part in oxidative metabolism. It may be useful to expand studies of fatty acids to cell types other than the fibroblasts and to species other than the 2 breeds of pigeons.

Several types of lipemia have been defined. Persons with one of these types—essential hypercholesteremia and hyperlipemia—are prone to athero-

Fig. 22. A. Vacuolization of rabbit aortic endothelial cells upon exposure to 650 μ of nicotine for 24 hours. Culture, 5 days old. Giemsa stain (×600). *B.* Explosive cytolysis of a rabbit aortic fibrocyte on entry into a current of nicotine solution (280 μg) injected into the perfusion chamber. Stop-motion, cinephotomicrography (×400).

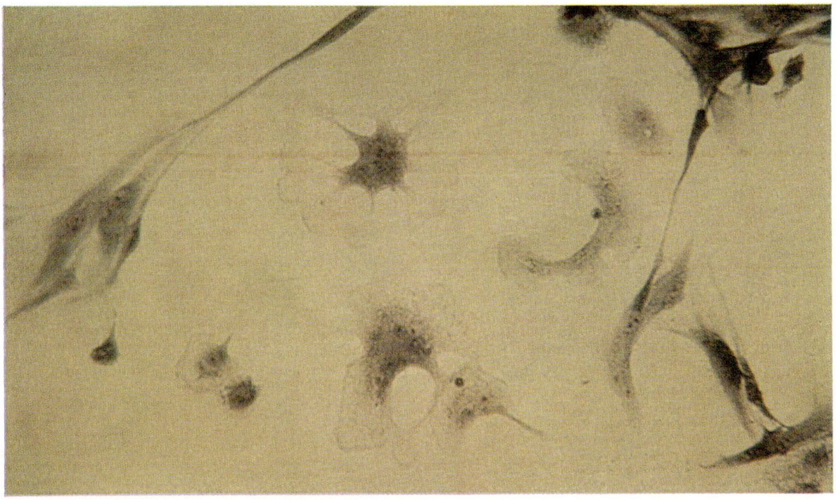

22 A

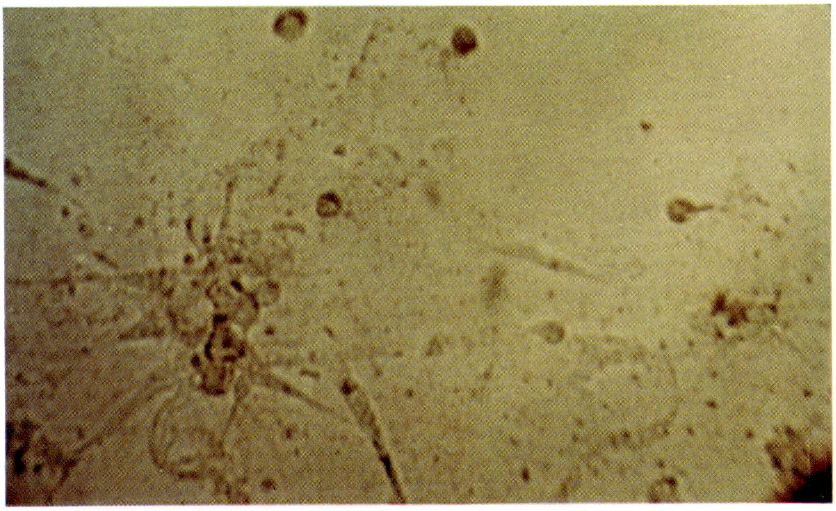

22 B

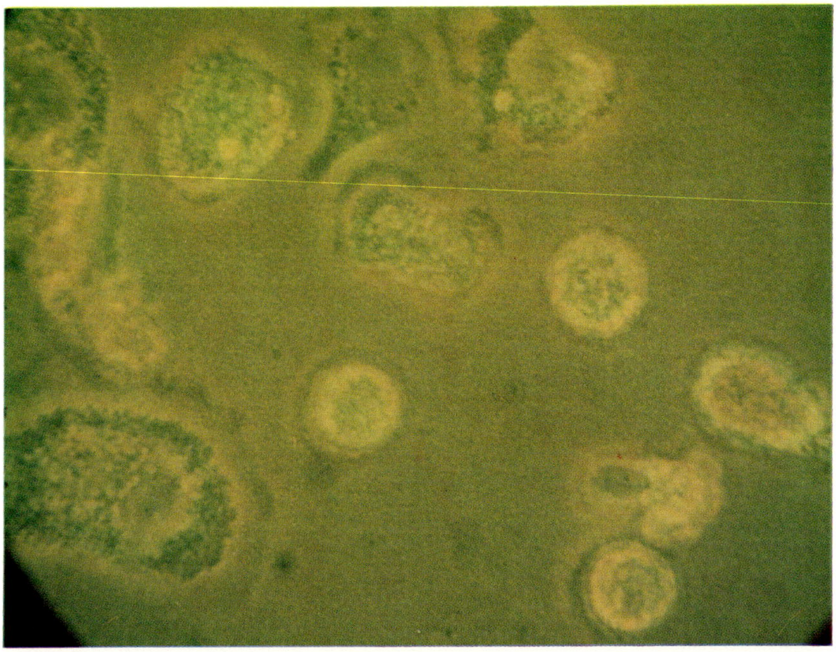

23 A

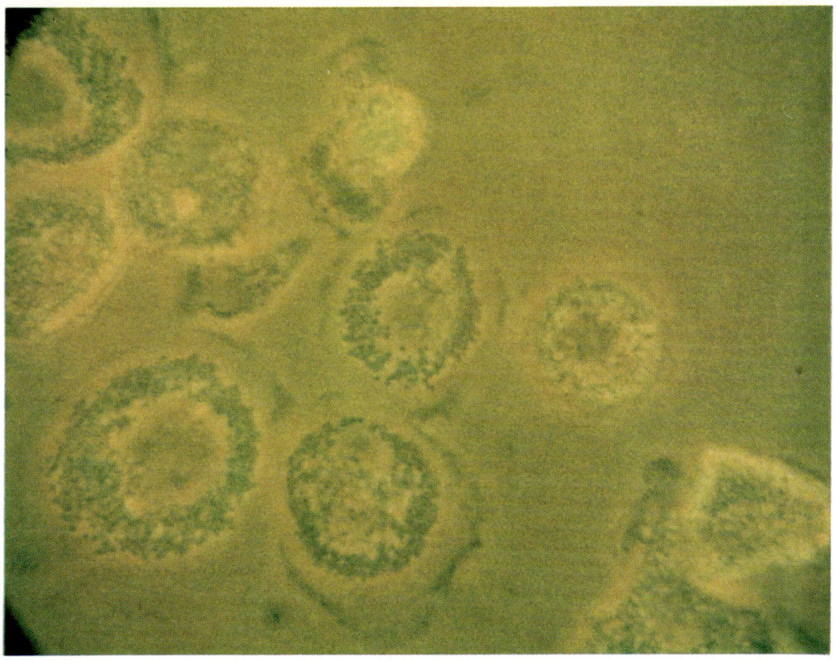

23 B

genesis. In pilot studies, SEEGER [1961] applied serum from a person with essential hypercholesteremia-hyperlipemia, obtained after various diets, mixed with normal serum or mixed with heparin, to cells in tissue cultures. A breakdown of triglycerides was observed. Due to a scarcity of materials, such studies are protracted and involved, but they seem to be worthwhile.

P. *Atherogenesis and in vitro Cultures*

1. General Comments

The elucidation of atherogenesis by tissue cultures has been attempted in several ways. Metabolic studies of nonvascular cells have contributed some information. Studies of whole arteries have been useful. Attempts have been made to produce 'atherosclerosis' *in vitro* by loading vascular cells with lipoids.

The culture of atherosclerotic arteries is one of the basic investigative approaches. Linked to such cultures are studies of the metabolism of cells grown from plaques, and reaction of such cells to chemicals, toxins, and microorganisms. The turnover of lipoids by cells grown from arteries has attracted much attention.

2. Formation of 'Foam Cells' *in vitro*

Arterial cells have been exposed to cholesterol solutions and suspensions, lipoprotein solutions, hypercholesteremic serum, and hyperlipemic serum. Loading of endothelial cells with lipoid has been successful. Results with fibroblasts have been erratic. The spontaneous accumulation of lipoids in fibroblasts has been overlooked. There is no doubt that the uptake of lipoids by endothelial cells exceeds the uptake by fibroblasts. The process is reversible—at least in part—upon removal of lipoids from the nutrient. According to LAZZARINI [1959], human aortic endothelial cells needed 50 μg of cholesterol per ml of nutrient to transform into 'foam cells', whereas coro-

---

Fig. 23. Early cell populations from rabbit aortae. *A.* Endothelial cells (left) and fat-laden macrophages (right) from aorta with plaques. *B.* Endothelial cells, only, from intact aorta. Reverse phase contrast, stop-motion, cinephotomicrography ($\times$ 500).

nary artery endothelial cells required 150 μg to 200 μg/ml. This observation has not received sufficient attention. Cells from different anatomic sites should be studied with regard to uptake of nonlabeled lipoids, radioactively labeled lipoids, and ability to synthesize lipoids. MURATA [1968] incubated 1-week-old chicken aortic endothelial cells for 3 days in MEM with 10% human lipemic serum, and transformed them into cells which resembled the 'foam cells' of chicken atherosclerotic arteries.

3. Culture of Atherosclerotic Tissues

No attention was paid to the composition of cell populations from atherosclerotic arteries in the course of metabolic studies by LAZZARINI [1959 and on]. References have been made to endothelial cells by LAZZARINI [1961b, 1962b, 1963a] in the course of study of canine atherosclerotic aortae and of dog and swine prostheses.

The cells form intact and atherosclerotic aortae of rabbits were described by POLLAK *et al.* [1960] and by KOKUBU [1961 and on]. The differences between the earliest cell outgrowth and growth curves from the 2 types of explants were significant (fig. 1). They were attributed to the variances in the dormancy of endothelial cells and fibroblasts, and to the presence of fat-laden cells in cultures from plaques. (figs. 23A and B). KASAI and POLLAK [1964] observed that the smooth muscle cells from rabbit aortae with plaques appeared 2 to 3 days later than that from explants of intact aortae. This was ascribed to the increased distance of muscle cells from the intimal surface caused by the intimal-subintimal thickening of the altered sector. No morphologic differences between corresponding cell types from the 2 sources were seen. There were only rare 'foam cells' visible in preparations from intact arteries, but many in preparations from plaques. Differences in amino acid metabolism and in the resistance to cytotoxins between cells from normo- and hypercholesteremic rabbits have been referred to in previous chapters.

Experimental lesions were also studied by WEXLER and THOMAS [1967]. Female virgin and breeder rats and male rats were used. Explants from altered aortic sectors—especially from the abdominal aorta—yielded fewer positive cultures, with fewer cells, at retarded growth rates, than explants from intact aortae. The cell population consisted of fibroblasts and a few smooth muscle cells. No endothelial cells and no fat-laden cells were seen. The seeming contradiction with the results of KOKUBU [1961 and on] is not realistic. Rat lesions are fibrous, without fat-laden cells. In the rabbit aortic culture, the large number of fat-laden macrophages and endothelial cells accounted for a steep and high growth curve.

Human aortae, and popliteal, femoral and tibial arteries with varying degrees of atherosclerosis were used by POLLAK and ADACHI [1968] for tissue cultures. Cells grown from intact and atherosclerotic human tissues did not differ morphologically. In pilot studies, they did not differ enzymatically. The more complicated the lesion, the poorer the culture results. About 10% of the culture attempts failed completely. Endothelial cells grew in 60%, fibrocytes in 90%, but myocytes in only 4% of the positive cultures. Fat-laden cells were never seen in cultures from complicated lesions or purely fibrous plaques. Harvest of macrophages was not abundant from yellow plaques, in sharp contrast to the 100% yield for rabbit aortic plaques. The topography of fat-laden cells, as described by POLLAK [1953a], may be used to explain the differences: *In vivo*, the rabbit's round (spheric) cells are seated between normal endothelial cells, often protruding into the lumen, and sometimes above the row of endothelial cells. This location is responsible for the easy detaching of these cells (fig. 24A). In man, fat-laden cells are polyhedric (they become spheric *in vitro*), wedged between or beneath the normal endothelial cells (fig. 24B). Fat-laden cells from rabbit aortic plaques are seen *in vitro* within 24 hours, but human fat-laden cells have not been seen before the 9th culture day. *In vitro*, human macrophages are smaller than those of rabbits, and have a less coarse granular cytoplasm and fewer cytoplasmic projections, according to POLLAK and ADACHI [1968].

4. Cellular Lipoids

At comparable oxygen concentration, uptake of labeled lipoprotein by cells from human and canine atherosclerotic aortae was 65 to 78% and 63 to 77.4% higher than uptake by cells from normal aortae, according to LAZZARINI [1961b, 1961d, 1961e, 1962b]. Uptake of protein-bound cholesterol by cells from canine homografts which had been in the hosts for 27 months was 2 to 38% higher than that of cells from normal or from atherosclerotic dog aortae. Plastic prosthesis of pigs had 48.6% higher uptake of H^3-serum-bound lipoprotein than host intima, according to LAZZARINI [1963a].

In contrast, it was found by LAZZARINI [1962a] that cells from normal aortae synthesized 40% more cholesterol from Na acetate-1-C^{14} than cells from atherosclerotic aortae. Using aqueous cholesterol-4-^{14}C, cholesterol-

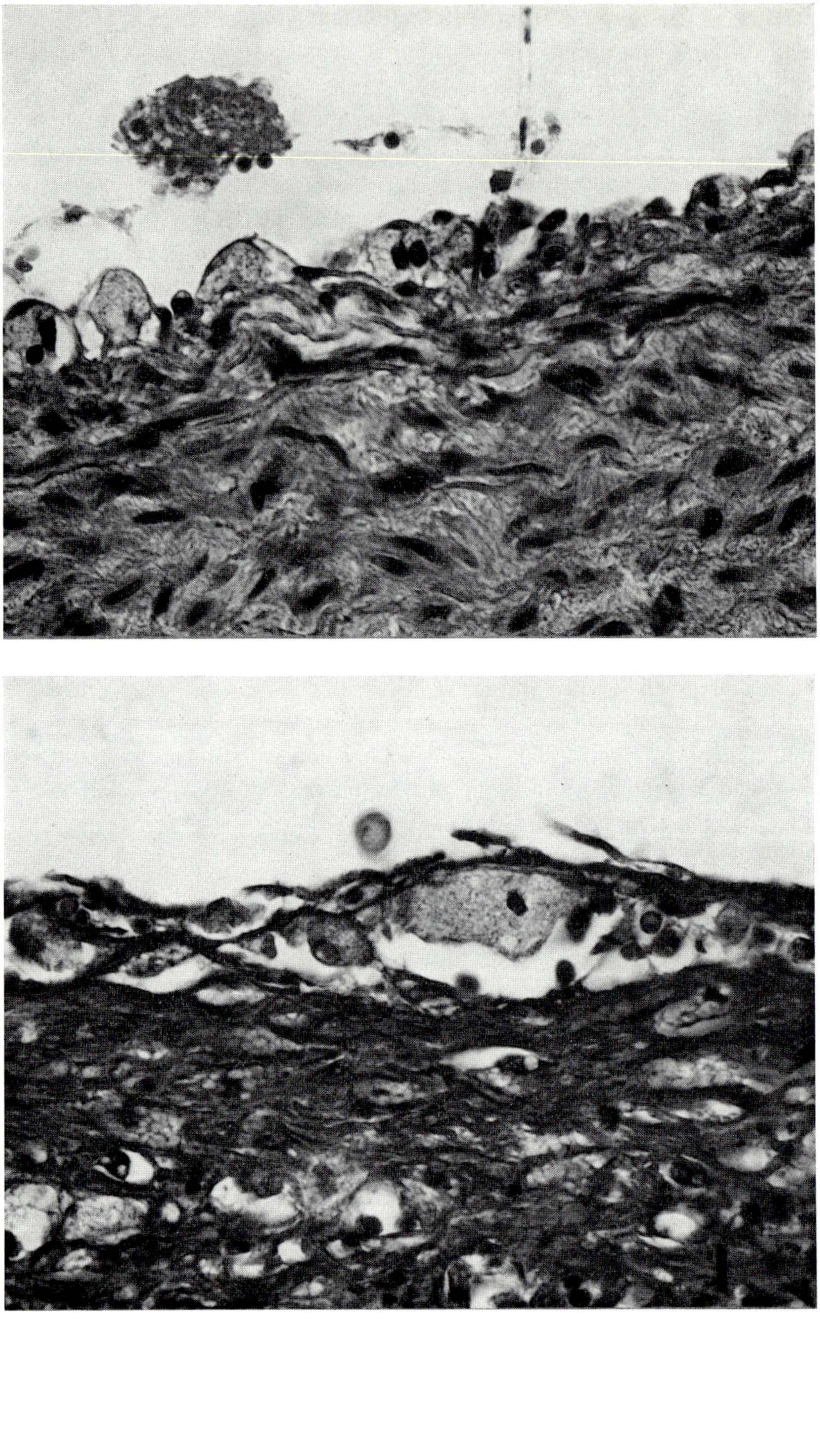

A

B

17-α-^{3}H, and cholesterol-26-^{14}C, Robertson [1965a] observed a 65 to 79% higher uptake by microsomal fractions from atherosclerotic plaques than by cells from intact aortae. Robertson [1968] explained his results in terms of the higher oxygen consumption of cells from atherosclerotic lesions. However, pertinent reports on the respiration of normal and atherosclerotic arterial tissues are conflicting. The intense cytochemical reaction of normal aortic endothelial cells to succinic dehydrogenase, and the weak reaction of lipoid-laden cells was considered by Lazzarini [1963a] as support of his concept. However, Koide and Pollak [1963] and Kasai and Pollak [1964] demonstrated a strong reaction for SDH in fat-laden macrophages from rabbit aortae (figs. 10D and 16C).

Murata [1968] prepared 'foam cells' by incubating 1-week-old chicken aortic cells for 3 days in MEM with 10% human lipemic serum. To such loaded cells, C^{14}-4-cholesterol, 0.1 μc/ml, was added. After 2, 4, and 6 hours of incubation, the transport rates for the fat-laden cells was 44 to 54% ($p < 0.001$) less than for the control cells. Murata [1968] also added 6 μc of H^{3}-7-α-cholesterol per ml of Puck's nutrient to endothelial cells and fibroblasts from aortae of *Macaca mulatta*, for 12 hours. The amount of H^{3} granules in the autoradiograms of cells from atherosclerotic aortae was negligible compared with the cells from the normal control aortae.

Fig. 24. A. Location of fat-laden cells in and above the endothelial layer of the rabbit aorta. Tissue section. Hematoxylin-eosin stain (×470). *B.* Location of fat-laden cells beneath the endothelial layer of the human aorta. Tissue section. Hematoxylin-eosin stain (×580).

V. CELL AGGREGATION

1. *In vitro*

About 150 reports on aggregation of embryonic cells from various sources into organ chimærae under special *in vitro* culture conditions have been listed by MOSCONA [1965]. Additional studies have been made since, but none have dealt with vascular cells.

The grouping of rabbit and human aortic smooth muscle cells into cell cords was described by KASAI and POLLAK [1964] (fig. 5) and also the spreading of smooth muscle cells beneath a layer of fibroblasts, imitating the architecture of the arterial wall (fig. 6). No attempt has been made to study the reaggregation of dispersed vascular cells—embryonic or adult—*in vitro*.

2. *In vivo*

Rat aortic fibroblasts were cultured for about 4 months, and over 15 generations were grown, by PRIEST and PRIEST [1964]. *In vitro* collagen production by these cells was proven by the presence of large amounts of hydroxyprolin in the nutrient. Millipore chambers were constructed using a plexiglass dish, 2.5 cm in diameter and 0.3 cm deep, covered by filter paper with a 0.22 μ pore size. Two chambers with 0.25 ml nutrient containing 5×10^5 cells, were implanted in the peritoneal cavity of the rats. After 3 weeks, blank capsules contained a plasma-like fluid. In the capsules with cells, 6 to 10 layers of fibroblasts were found, within an intercellular substance which stained as collagen and which, in electronmicrographs, appeared as fibers with the 640 Å periodicity characteristic of collagen. A fibrous coat developed around the capsule. Upon hydrolysis, this coat yielded a positive reaction for hydroxyprolin. The authors suggested that this material is the product of fibroblasts within the chambers. There is no doubt that the ability of rat aortic fibroblasts to produce collagen persists both *in vitro* and *in vivo*.

Small Millipore chambers, constructed of a plastic ring and 2 filter papers, were used by GONZALES [1963a, 1963b] to study the reaction of white blood cells to hypercholesteremia. A buffy coat with blood leukocytes from normocholesteremic rabbits was introduced into the chambers which were implanted subcutaneously into the host rabbits fed a cholesterol diet for 3 to 6 weeks. Leukocytes within the chambers transformed into 'foam cells' and stained positively for lipoids, lipase, acid phosphomonoesterase, esterase, and mucopolysaccharides.

WADA and POLLAK [1967a] and POLLAK and WADA [1968a] set out to study the transformation of various arterial and venous cells into 'foam cells' *in vivo*. The inability of the investigators to clone smooth muscle cells led to the use of mixed cell populations over 3 weeks old. Samples were checked for the presence of endothelial cells, fibrocytes and myocytes, but no attempt was made to determine the numbers of each cell type. Trypsinized cells, dispersed in physiologic saline solution, were counted. Since 0.3 ml of suspension was to be introduced into each chamber, the number of cells was adjusted to 5,000–10,000/0.3 ml. Control chambers were filled with 0.3 ml of saline solution. Each chamber was constructed from a plastic ring 2 mm high, 15 mm in outside diameter, and 10 mm in inside diameter, to which 2 Millipore filter papers of 0.45 μ pore size and 13.9 mm diameter were attached by cement. The cell suspension was injected through a hole in the plastic ring, and the hole was sealed with nylon thread.

Multiple chambers were implanted subcutaneously along the spine into serologically compatible litter mates of the donor rabbits. The host rabbits were divided into 2 groups. One group was fed rabbit chow, while the other was fed chow, 1 egg yolk, and 1 g of powdered cholesterol each day. The blood cholesterol of the 1st group averaged 85 mg/100 ml throughout the experiment; that of the cholesterol-fed group rose to an average of 1,640 mg/100 ml in 3 weeks. At that point, the cholesterol averaged 312 mg/100 ml in control diffusion chambers without cells.

The dispersion of cells was checked on the 3rd day in one of the chambers. Multiple clusters of cells were seen (fig. 25A). After 3 weeks, there was a distinct reaggregation of aortic cells. More or less uniformly wide bands had formed, consisting of a broad central part, with many elongated cells, and a surface layer of endothelial cells (fig. 25B). The broad layer stained characteristically for muscle. Myocytes and fibrocytes were present. Collagen could be demonstrated by special stains. Elastic fibers were not visualized. In some aggregates, there were whirle-like formations, with abundant collagen and chondroblasts. No ossification was seen after 3 weeks of observation. Fat-laden cells were seen on the surface of thickened portions of the aggregates in hypercholesteremic hosts.

Admittedly, it takes imagination to identify the aggregates as primitive aortae. Possibly, more perfect chimærae would be obtained if embryonic aortic cell cultures were used for the experiments. However, cells *in vitro* may undergo reversal to an immature stage; the *in vivo* aggregates are reminiscent of embryonic tissues, even though adult cells were introduced. Injection of cell suspensions which would include fat-laden macrophages would be useful. One could attempt to influence the reaggregation of aortic cells by injecting various chemicals, into the diffusion chambers, or by hormone treatment of host animals. The phenomenon is not typical for aortic cells. Chimæric *in vivo* reaggregation of adrenal, cardiac, and corneal cells has been demonstrated by Pollak and Wada [1968a] and Wada and Pollak [1969].

The observation of *in vivo* reaggregation of aortic cells was a chance finding. The question of transformation of various vascular cells into 'foam cells' could be only partly answered. No fat-laden cells were seen in the suspensions before they were injected into the diffusion chambers. On the removal of the aggregates and their transfer to *in vitro* nutrient, there was a marked difference in the character of the populations, when aggregates and cells removed from normo- and from hypercholesteremic rabbits were compared. After 7 days, only a few macrophages were seen in cultures from aggregates removed from normocholesteremic hosts. Nearly two-thirds of the cells were fibrocytes and nearly one-third were endothelial cells (fig. 25 C). In 7-day-old cultures from aggregates removed from hypercholesteremic rabbits, nearly two-thirds of the cell population were fat-laden macrophages, with the rest being fibrocytes and a few endothelial cells (fig. 25 D).

Fig. 25. A. Rabbit aortic cells retrieved from a diffusion chamber 3 days after it had been implanted into a host rabbit. May-Grünwald-Giemsa stain (×450). *B.* Rabbit aortic cells aggregated into a rudimentary aorta within a diffusion chamber 3 weeks after it had been implanted into a host rabbit. Hematoxylin-eosin stain (×90). *C. In vitro* cell population 7 days after transfer of an *in vivo* aortic aggregate from a chamber removed from a normocholesteremic rabbit. Unstained (×25). *D. In vitro* cell population 7 days after transfer of an *in vivo* aortic aggregate from a chamber removed from a hypercholesteremic rabbit. Unstained (×25). A, B and C correspond to figures 2, 1 and 4 in Wada, A. and Pollak, O.J. [1967a].

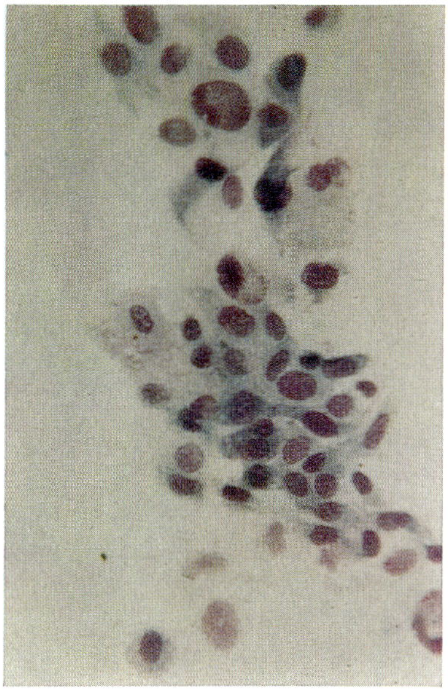

25 A

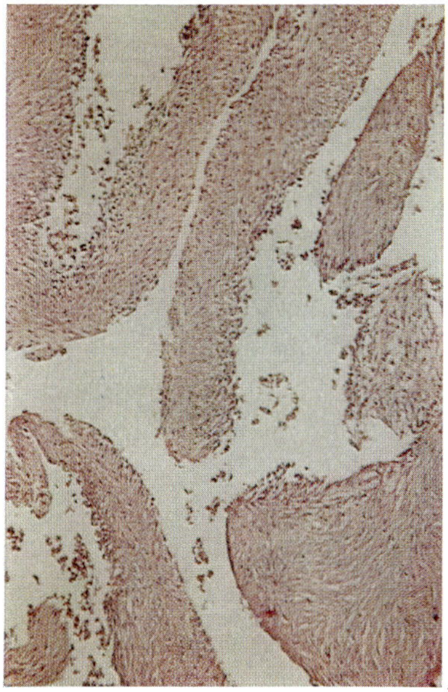

25 B

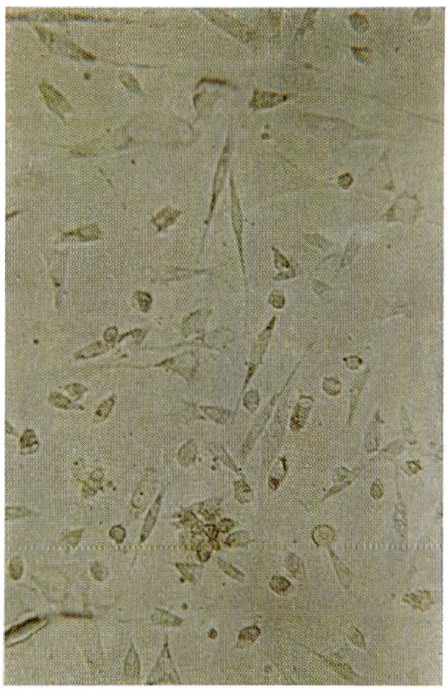

25 C

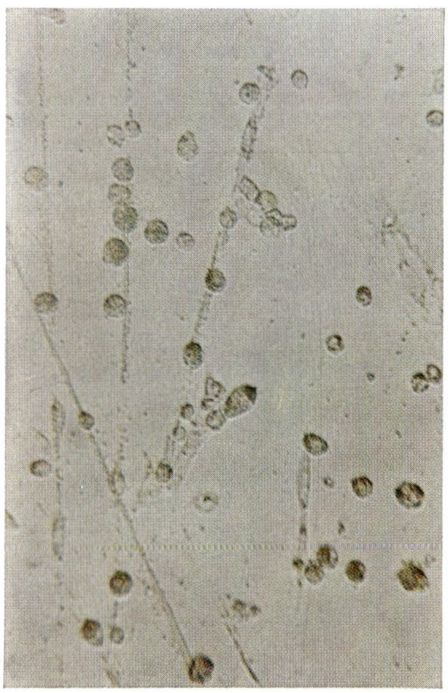

25 D

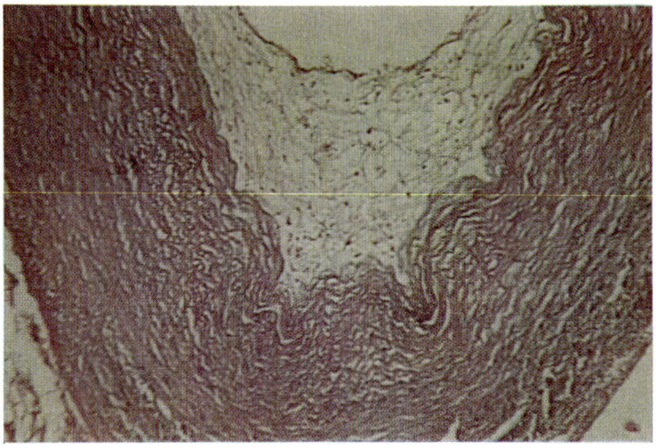

26 A

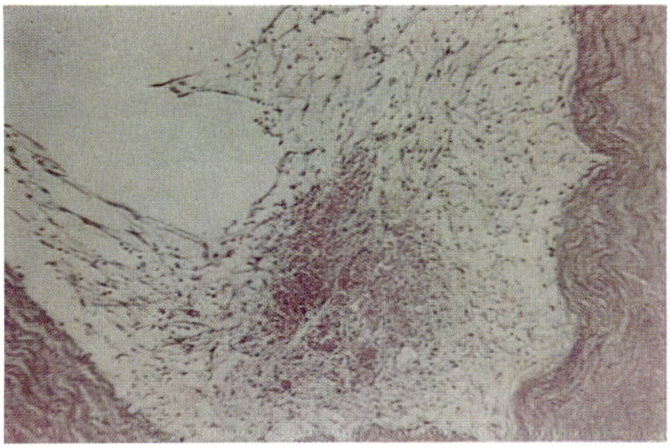

26 B

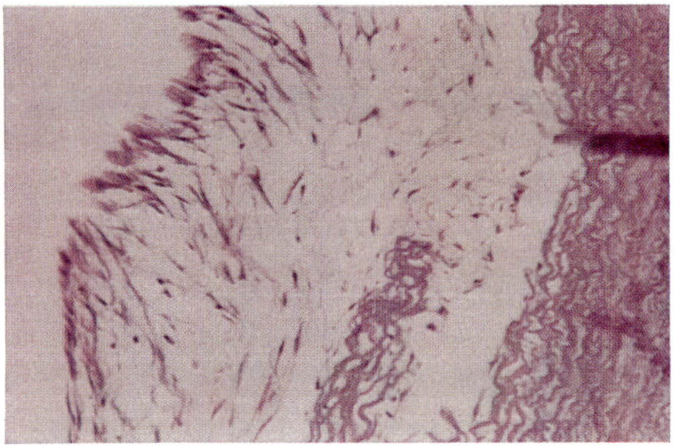

26 C

VI. *IN VIVO* VASCULAR TISSUE CULTURES

1. Ocular Implants

Cell growth on the inner surface of synthetic prosthesis, on dacron hubs suspended in arteries, and along pulsating tubes implanted into animals may be referred to as *in vivo* cell culture. Truly, the first attempt to grow arterial tissues in the living animal was made by HIGGINBOTHAM [1957a] and by HIGGINBOTHAM and HIGGINBOTHAM [1958]. Rabbit aortic explants were placed in the anterior eye chamber of host rabbits. Three drops of 0.5% tetracaine HCl solution were used to anesthesize the cornea. A 3 to 4 mm incision was made at the corneoscleral junction and the aortic explant was pushed into the chamber, with the intima facing outward. The results were unaffected by differences in the age of donor and host, but uniformity was affected when donor and host were of opposite sex.

The adventitia of the homotransplant became attached to the iris in less than 8 days. The intima of normal aortic implants remained translucent and reflected the light even after 8 months. The thickened intima of atherosclerotic implants became extensively vascularized by vessels from the iris within 30 days. Histologically, transplants of normal aortae had not changed, except that the smooth muscle cells had assumed a vertical position to the intimal surface. In transplants from atherosclerotic aortae, 'foam cells' appeared, the elastica was split, and cholesterol ester crystals were present.

HIGGINBOTHAM [1957b] observed a decrease in the number of fat-laden cells and in the degree of sudanophilia in atheromatous implants. A fibro-

---

Fig. 26. A. In vivo reaction of a noneverted aortic ring-segment 3 weeks after implantation in a diffusion chamber in a host rabbit. Hematoxylin-eosin stain (× 50). *B. In vivo* reaction of a noneverted aortic ring-segment 4 weeks after implantation in a diffusion chamber in a host rabbit. Hematoxylin-eosin stain (× 50). *C. In vitro* outgrowth of endothelial cells after transfer of a noneverted aortic ring-segment kept for 3 weeks *in vivo* in a diffusion chamber in a normocholesteremic host. Culture, 3 days old. Hematoxylin-eosin stain (× 100). A, B and C correspond to figures 2, 4 and 6 in WADA, A. and POLLAK, O.J. [1967b].

elastic cap formed, the internal elastica reduplicated, clefts of free cholesterol crystals appeared between the cells after 4 months, and persisted for 8 to 16 months, while cholesterol ester crystals slowly disappeared. Sudanophilia, which originally had been diffuse, was then seen only in necrotic areas around the crystals. Calcification was noted. The formation of a cap over the lesion, and other changes, were interpreted as evidence of regression. They could be interpreted as evidence of the organization of 'foam cell' plaques. There is ample room for expansion of this experimental model.

2. Initiation of Atherogenesis

a) General Comments

The localization of atherosclerotic lesions is one of the puzzles of atherogenesis. The rate of progression and ultimate limit of atherogenesis are also puzzling. The character of atherogenesis is fairly typical for each species: Experimental lesions develop in the same location in which spontaneous lesions are found. The start and the course of atherogenesis are, however, not governed by identical factors.

In some species (including the rabbit) the first visible lesions are seen in the ascending aorta, while lesions in the terminal aorta appear last. A similar gradient as that for the appearance of lesions has been observed for the transmural passage of albumin, cholesterol, and lipoproteins *in vivo* and *in vitro* (cf. III. B). Differences in lipoid composition and synthesis were reported by RABINOWITZ and RIEMENSCHNEIDER [1961] and differences in free amino acid composition of various aortic sectors were noted by ENGEL and POLLAK [1961a]. With plaque formation in the proximal aorta, shifts in amino acids were recorded by ENGEL and POLLAK [1961b] and, similarly, shifts of certain enzymes to the distal parts by MAIER and HAIMOVICI [1965].

Disturbances of the blood flow, and other rheological and physical factors, play an important role in the formation and localization of advanced lesions. To HAIMOVICI and MAIER [1966], the most important factor in the initiation of atherogenesis is local susceptibility, demonstrated by experiments in which aortic and pulmonary artery sectors were interchanged.

b) Subcutaneous Implants

To assign proper weights to various factors, and on the assumption that local tissue avidity for cholesterol may be one of the most important agents,

POLLAK and WADA [1966, 1967b, 1968c], WADA and POLLAK [1967] and POLLAK [1967] studied rabbit aortic tissues within subcutaneously implanted diffusion chambers. Ring-shaped aortic segments, 1.5 mm to 2 mm high, were placed in Millipore chambers. These were constructed in the same manner as in *in vivo* aggregation experiments (cf. V. 2). Chambers of double height, 4 mm, were made by fusing 2 plastic rings. Rings without holes were used, since the chambers were closed following the insertion of aorta. Control chambers contained 0.5 ml of saline solution, without tissues. Serologically compatible litter mates were used as donors and recipients, respectively—to minimize the chance of rejection. No attention was paid to the sex of the rabbits. The animals were adults, 2.7 kg to 3.5 kg weight. The chambers were implanted along the spine in such a manner that the sequence followed the position of the segments in the donor rabbit. Up to 20 chambers were implanted into 1 host. The chambers were removed after 2, 3, 4, or 5 weeks. One series of rabbits was kept on a basic diet of Purina chow; the other series received the chow and a daily supplement of 1 fried egg yolk and 1 g of cholesterol (Merck).

The blood cholesterol of the control rabbits remained fairly stable, about 85 mg/100 ml. Within the diffusion chambers, the cholesterol was between 74 mg and 96 mg/100 ml. The blood cholesterol of the experimental animals rose, in weekly intervals, from 85 mg/100 ml to 495 mg/100 ml, 1,350 mg/100 ml, 1,643 mg/100 ml, and 2,950 mg/100 ml. The cholesterol within the chambers rose, too, but it was consistently lower than in the blood. In chambers with aortic explants, there was a rise in cholesterol during the first 2 weeks, followed by a decline. The deficit was accompanied by an increase in tissue cholesterol. After the 3rd week, the chamber-fluid cholesterol was 25% less than in chambers without tissue; after 4 weeks, it was 27% less, and after 5 weeks, it was 69% less.

Noneverted aortic rings reacted *in vivo* by distinct broadening of the subendothelial layer. The subintima pushed an intact endothelium toward the center of the lumen, either in the shape of a crescent, or later in the shape of a ring, with subsequent reduction in the size of the lumen (fig. 26A). (WEXLER and THOMAS [1967] noted a similar reaction in *in vitro* cultures of rat aortic rings.) At first, the number of cells in the subendothelial collagenous matter was small. Fibrocytes and, possibly, myocytes were present. Later, the cellularity increased, sometimes with a focal center which became vascularized (fig. 26B). Within the capillaries there were a few blood cells. (This observation brought to mind two reports of CLARK *et al.* [1931] and CLARK and CLARK [1939] on new blood-vessel formation in as short a time as 6 days in tissues within chambers implanted in rabbit ears.) Upon transfer of such aortic tissue from diffusion chambers into an *in vitro* culture, a fern-like outgrowth of endothelial cells was seen above the thickened subendothelial layer (fig. 26C).

Adventitial proliferation paralleled that of the subendothelial growth of noneverted ring-segments. This resulted in limitation of the observation period. After 5 weeks, the whole aortic implant was encased in a rubbery gelatinous matter. (There was a striking similarity with the report made by PRIEST and PRIEST [1964] on the reaction around intraperitoneally-implanted chambers with fibroblasts.)

Entirely different results were obtained by WADA and POLLAK [1967] with everted aortic ring-segments. After 2 weeks, the endothelium had either patchy edema (fig. 27A), or patchy thickening with up to 5 tiers of cells (fig. 27B). After 3 weeks, at a time when the control chambers contained at least 300 mg/100 ml cholesterol, intimal-subintimal lipoid cushions were seen (fig. 27C). (In cholesterol-fed rabbits, similar plaques developed when the blood cholesterol reached 300 mg/100 ml, according to POLLAK [1945].) As in feeding experiments, intimal plaques developed more often in segments from the ascending aorta than in distal segments. Upon transfer of implants with lesions to *in vitro* cultures, many fat-laden macrophages were harvested.

c) Trauma and Atherogenesis

WADA and POLLAK [1967] endeavored to explain the differences in the fate of noneverted and everted aortic ring-segments *in vivo*. Mechanical trauma in the process of everting the ring—pulling and stretching—resulted in microfractures of the aortic intima. Interplay between the trauma and the intrachamber cholesterol caused intramural deposit of sudanophilic material. In these experiments, the trauma preceded the presence of cholesterol within the chambers. It has long been known that trauma promotes insudation of lipoids into the arterial intima, when it precedes hypercholesteremia or when it occurs in a subject with preexisting hypercholesteremia. It has also

---

Fig. 27. In vivo reaction of everted aortic ring-segments in hypercholesteremic rabbits. *A.* Intimal endothelial edema, 2 weeks after implantation of the diffusion chamber. Hematoxylin-eosin stain (× 500). *B.* Intimal endothelial proliferation, 2 weeks after implantation of the diffusion chamber. Hematoxylin-eosin stain (× 250). *C.* Intimal lipoid cushion—plaque, 3 weeks after implantation of the diffusion chamber. Hematoxylin-eosin stain (× 125). B and C correspond to figures 7 and 8 in WADA, A. and POLLAK, O.J. [1967b].

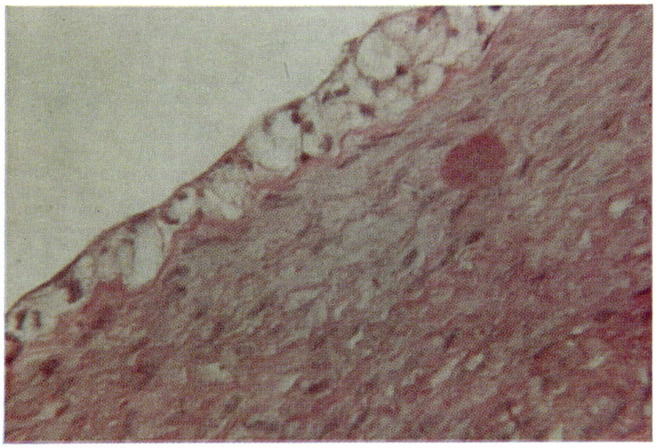

27 *A*

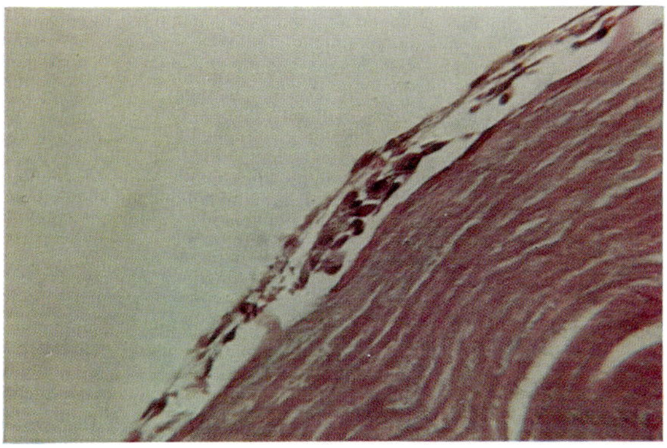

27 *B*

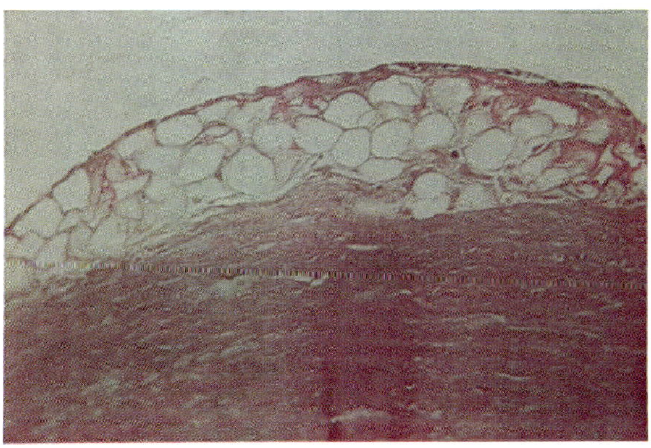

27 *C*

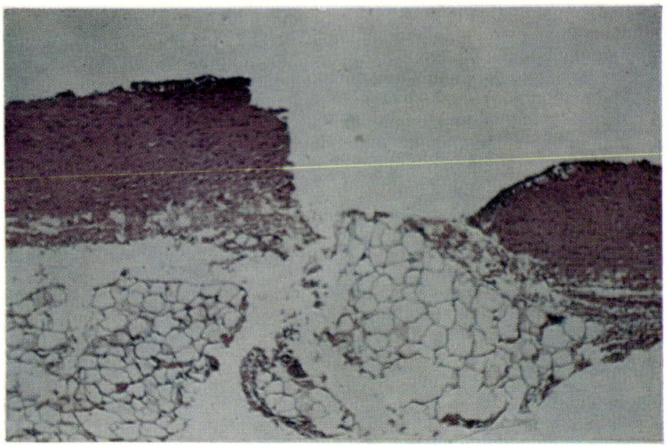

28 A

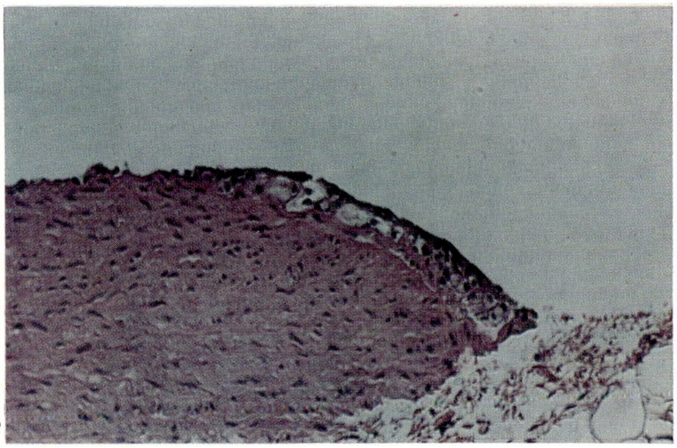

28 B

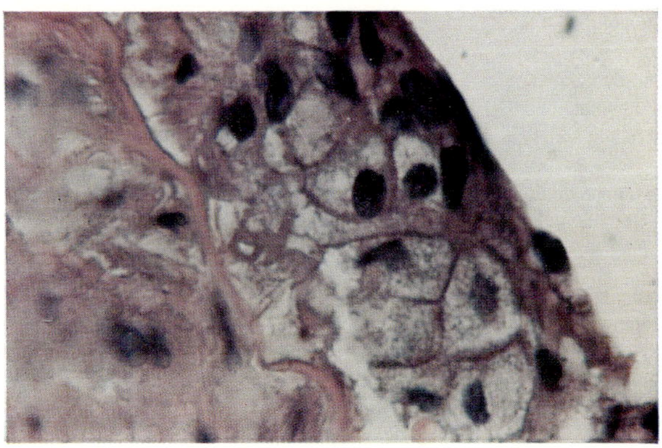

28 C

been established that trauma may be mechanical—such as in the described experiments—or of other physical or chemical nature. (POLLAK [1965] referred to the fact that the literature abounds with reports on the initiation and promotion of atherogenesis by puncturing the arterial wall, applying extreme heat or cold, administering macromolecular substances, bacterial toxins, various hormones, pressure amines, etc.) Cholesterol may be the most important lipoid deposited in the arterial wall but it certainly is not the only one.

To strengthen the concept of the triad—artery, trauma, cholesterol—as initiating atherogenesis, POLLAK [1968] and POLLAK and WADA [1968b] cut the wall of noneverted aortic ring-segments before placing them into diffusion chambers for implantation. Within 2 weeks after implantation endothelial edema was seen, and within 3 weeks plaques developed on the shoulders of the gap caused by the incision (fig. 28).

The position of the plaques was quite similar to that seen on cross-sectioning of the ostia of vertebral arteries of children and young adults. The location of such plaques has been often ascribed to rheologic factors. In the experiments in which extracirculatory atherogenesis has been produced within diffusion chambers, all rheologic factors have been eliminated. No formed blood elements were present, and there was no clotting. The artery was the parietal factor, and the cholesterol was the humoral factor. Trauma acted as a complement, or mediating factor. The sequence of the intimal reaction was endothelail edema and proliferation, and 'foam cell plaque' formation.

In the experiments of WADA and POLLAK [1967b], insudation of intercellular fluid with cholesterol occurred after cell proliferation. This was documented by the appearance of tissue sudanophilia and by the cholesterol deficit within chambers with implants. The sequence might be different if the chambers with aortic rings were implanted in a host animal with severe hypercholesteremia. It would lead to a speedier accumulation of cholesterol within the chambers. The formula of trauma—aortic reaction—cholesterol insudation seems simple enough. However, the fluid which seeps into the chamber, contains not only cholesterol but also all the other constituents of

---

Fig. 28. A–C. In vivo intimal 'foam cell' plaques on the shoulders of a cut through a noneverted aortic ring-segment, developed 3 weeks after implantation in a diffusion chamber in a hypercholesteremic rabbit. Hematoxylin-eosin stain (*A.* ×50; *B.* ×150; *C.* ×500).

blood plasma—though in great dilutions—such as lipfanogens and hormones. On detailed analysis, the phenomenon may yet prove quite complicated.

d) Intraperitoneal Implants

The distribution of plaques in the rabbit aortae is patchy, and the size of the plaques is small. Thus, the detection of lesions in aortic ring-segments within implanted chambers is left to chance. POLLAK [1969] and POLLAK and WADA [1968c] placed whole rabbit aortae into DeBakey's crimpled dacron tubing, 1 cm in diameter, such as that used for the prosthesis of iliac human arteries. Such 15 cm long pieces of tubing were sealed on both ends with Millipore filter paper, 1 cm in diameter and 0.45 μ pore size. The aorta was secured in position by nylon sutures at each end. The development of cholesterol-atherosclerosis in aortae implanted into rabbits on a cholesterol-rich diet could be observed and could be compared with the lesions which had developed in the host's aorta. The difference between hypercholesteremia of the host and the cholesterol level within the tubing accounted for the much less severe atherosclerosis in the implanted aorta than in the host's aorta. The differences were quantitative. The distribution of sudanophilia in the implant was the same as in the host aorta.

These were pilot studies. Obviously, many variations on these experiments may be foreseen. A donor's aorta could be split longitudinally, with one half implanted in a normocholesteremic host and the other in a hypercholesteremic host. Aortae of hypercholesteremic rabbits, with experimental lesions, could be placed within tubing in normocholesteremic rabbits to investigate the possibility of lesion regression. This experimental model also lends itself to therapeutic trials. The studies could be expanded to many species.

VII. REVIEW

It seems appropriate to conclude this text with a summary of achievements, and look toward the future of this discipline. Many questions were raised in the introductory chapter concerning various aspects of atherogenesis. Elucidation of the initial and early phases of atherogenesis on the cellular level seems feasible. Indeed, some questions have been answered during the first decade of this research approach. But many more remain unanswered, either for lack of time, lack of interest or support, or because of faulty experiment design.

In the author's opinion, these are the highlights of the first years of vascular tissue culture research:

1. Three distinct cell types have been identified in vascular cultures from several species: endothelial cells, fibrocytes, and myocytes.

2. A fourth cell type, the fat-laden macrophage, has been identified in preparations from atherosclerotic arteries of rabbit and man.

3. The question of the origin of the so-called 'foam cell' has yet to be answered satisfactorily. The transformation of intimal endothelial cells into fat-laden cells seems certain. The possibility that myocytes may transform into such cells has neither been proved nor disproved. The question could be answered by *in vivo* experiments with pure cell lines cultured *in vitro*.

4. The fact that most metabolic studies have been done with aortic fibroblasts and endothelial cells, or a mixture of the two, is the biggest limitation in the evaluation of past tissue culture work. Past investigations should be repeated with smooth muscle cells, and all studies should be expanded to explants from blood vessels which are less prone to atherogenesis than aortae.

5. The production of mucopolysaccharides by vascular cells needs further investigation, particularly with regard to the sequence of the production of polysaccharides and the accumulation of lipoids.

6. The role of fibrocytes and of myocytes in the production of ground substance and elastic fibers has yet to be studied. Smooth muscle cells have, so far, been studied morphologically only.

7. The enzyme activities of aortic cells have been studied only superficially. The correlation of cellular enzyme reactions with the results of histochemical and chemical tissue analysis may prove informative.

8. The investigation of amino acid turnover by cells from normal and atherosclerotic tissues has uncovered important differences. The studies should be extended to individual cell lines, to vascular cells from various species, and quantitative essays should be carried out.

9. The effect of various carbohydrates on lipoid turnover by vascular cells should be studied *in vitro*.

10. The regulation of the transmembrane transport of lipoids by anions and cations has been clarified, at least for human endothelial cells.

11. Cellular homeostasis, regulating the uptake of extracellular lipoids and the intracellular synthesis of lipoids, has been recorded.

12. Quantitative differences in lipoid synthesis by cells from normal arterial sectors and by cells from atherosclerotic sectors have been reported, with conflicting results. Repeating the pertinent studies with pure cell lines of various species, with particular attention paid to fat-laden macrophages, should produce uniform results.

13. The area of cytopharmacology is very open to further exploration. So far, attempts to influence lipoid deposits have been made only with fibroblasts. Experiments with saturated and unsaturated fatty acids have led to conflicting reports and reevaluation is warranted.

14. Cytotoxicologic studies have shown that hypercholesteremia increases the vulnerability of arterial cells to toxic matter.

15. The field of cytogenetics has not been explored although a study of arterial cells from two breeds of pigeons revealed significant differences in arachidonic acid. Recognition of the genetic regulation of enzyme pathways suggests many new research topics.

16. *In vitro* tissue cultures have many limitations. The cells lose their orientation toward the surface of tissues. They do not interact with adjacent cells or with remote cells. They are exposed to an artificial environment instead of a self-renewing intercellular fluid. The growth rate, morphologic appearance, and metabolism of cells *in vitro* may vary with the methodology of tissue culture. Culture results are influenced by the selection of explants. Cells of different types from mixed populations, pure cultures, and first or subsequent generations do not behave alike. Conformity of technique is a prerequisite for uniform results.

17. Supplementing *in vitro* cultures with animal experiments has been profitable. But many additional experiments are needed.

18. The aggregation of dispersed aortic cells *in vitro* has not been attempted. Reaggregation *in vivo* has been worthwhile. Again, additional investigation using embryonic cells and different cell populations is desirable. Hormones may influence the formation of chimæric aggregates. Hyaluronidase could prevent cell aggregation.

19. *In vivo* cultures led to the important conclusion that atherogenesis can be produced outside the circulatory system, in the absence of rheologic factors and clotting factors. Extension of this approach, by placing whole arteries into synthetic tubing, has been suggested.

20. New projects, in addition to those suggested can be devised.

In the introductory chapters, a stand had been taken against oversimplification of the problem of atherogenesis and for the multifactorial etiology. It now appears that the initiation of atherogenesis follows a simple formula: 'trauma' to the intima, reaction of a susceptible intima, and seepage of 'cholesterol' into the damaged intima.

The episodic character of atherogenesis accounts for the presence of different types of lesions. Trauma and cholesterol represent the two initiating agents. They provoke a characteristic tissue reaction—intimal endothelial edema, proliferation, and plaque formation. Many more factors, singly or in combination, simultaneously or in a sequence, promote the progression, control the speed, determine the ultimate degree, and cause complications in atherogenesis which lead to clinical manifestations. Attempts to prevent the clinical manifestations—the complications of anatomical alterations, to modify, slow down, or block the evolution of atherogenesis can be made at various stages of the disease process. The prevention of the earliest phase of atherogenesis seems most desirable. To achieve this, knowledge of the initiating factors is essential. To assign the proper weight to each atherogenic factor is a major challenge. The vascular tissue culture may have great usefulness in meeting this challenge.

REFERENCES

ADACHI, M.; ADACHI, T. and POLLAK, O.J.: Hypercholesteremia: Effect on the depression of tissue respiration by nicotine. J. amer. Geriat. Soc. *14:* 221–230 (1966).

AYKAN, T.B.: Comparative study of the metabolism of twenty two months old aortic and myocardial cultures of the rat. I. Morphological and growth characteristics. New Istanbul Contr. clin. Sci. *7:* 64–74 (1964).

BAILEY, J.M.: Lipid metabolism in cultured cells. I. Factors affecting cholesterol uptake. Proc. Soc. exp. Biol., N.Y. *107:* 30–35 (1961). – Lipid metabolism in cultured cells. III. Cholesterol excretion process. Amer. J. Physiol. *207:* 1221–1225 (1964). – Lipid metabolism in cultured cells. IV. Serum alpha globulins and cellular cholesterol exchange. Exp. Cell Res. *37:* 175–182 (1965). – Lipid metabolism in cultured cells. VI. Lipid biosynthesis in serum and synthetic growth media. Biochim. biophys. Acta *125:* 226–236 (1966). – Cellular lipid nutrition and lipid transport; in G.H. ROTHBLAT and D. KRITCHEVSKY, Lipid metabolism and tissue culture cells, pp. 85–109 (Wistar Inst. Symposium Monograph No. 6, 1967).

BAILEY, J.M.; GEY, G.O. and MAYMANDI-NEJAD, A.: Lipid metabolism in cultured cells. II. Cholesterol uptake from serum of normal and atherosclerotic human adults. Proc. Soc. exp. Biol., N.Y. *107:* 594–597 (1961).

BEHBEHANI, A.M.; MELNICK, J.L. and BAKEY, M.E. DE: Continuous cell strains derived from human atheromatous lesions and their viral susceptibility. Proc. Soc. exp. Biol., N.Y. *118:* 759–763 (1965).

BELLMAN, S.; BOSTRÖM, H.; GÖTHMAN, B. and RODMAN, L.: On the extracorporeal survival of aortic segments: Isotope and respiratory studies. Angiology, Baltimore *7:* 396–402 (1956).

BENCH, K.G.; KING, D.W. and SOCOLOW, E.L.: The sources of lipid accumulation in L-cells. J. biophys. biochem. Cytol. *9:* 135–139 (1961).

BENEWOLENSKAJA, S.W.: Hematopoiesis in cultures of the embryonic liver of men. Arch. exp. Zellforsch. *9:* 128–141 (1929).

BJORKSTEN, J.: A mechanism of cholesterol deposition on arterial walls. Proc. Soc. exp. Biol., N.Y. *81:* 350–353 (1952).

BLOOM, W.: Studies on fibers in tissue cultures. II. The development of elastic fibers in cultures of embryonic heart and aorta. Arch. Zellforsch. *9:* 6–13 (1929).

BRANWOOD, A.W.: Growth pattern of arterial endothelium in tissue culture and the effect of lipids, heparin and oestradiol on tissue cells. Unpublished. Cardiovascular Tissue Culture Conf., Dover, Del., USA (1961a). – Cardiovascular tissue culture: A new discipline in atherosclerosis research. J. Atheroscler. Res. *1:* 358–361 (1961b). – Modern concepts of the pathogenesis of coronary atherosclerosis, pp. 110–132 (Livingston, Edinburgh/London 1963).

BRIGGS, A.H. and MELVIN, S.: Ion movements in isolated rabbit aortic strips. Amer. J. Physiol. *201:* 365–368 (1961).

BURNS, D.A.: Low cost time-lapse cinephotomicrography. Amer. J. med. Sci. *248:* 697–702 (1964).

CAMERON, G. and CHAMBERS, R.: Neoplasm studies. III. Organization of cells of human tumors in tissue culture. Amer. J. Cancer *30:* 115–129 (1937).

CARREL, A. and BURROWS, M.T.: Cultivation of adult tissues and organs outside the body. J. amer. med. Ass. *55:* 1379–1381 (1910).

CASTOR, C.W.; PRINCE, R.K. and DORSTEWITZ, E.L.: Characteristics of human 'fibroblasts' cultivated *in vitro* from different anatomical sites. Lab. Invest. *11:* 703–713 (1962).

CATELLI, W.P.; NICKERSON, R.J.; NEWELL, J.M. and RUTSTEIN, D.D.: Serum NEFA following fat, carbohydrate and protein ingestion, and during fasting as related to intracellular lipid deposition. J. Atheroscler. Res. *6:* 328–341 (1966).

CHOBANIAN, A.V.: Sterol synthesis in the human arterial intima. J. clin. Invest. *47:* 595–603 (1968).

CHOI, B.H.; FLORENTIN, R.A. and LEE, S.K.: Damaging effect of hypercholesterolemic swine serum in tissue culture. Fed. Proc. *27:* 575 (1968).

CLARK, E.R. and CLARK, E.L.: Microscopic observations on the growth of capillaries in the living animal. Amer. J. Anat. *64:* 251–302 (1939).

CLARK, E.R.; HITSCHLER, H.T.; KIRBY-SMITH, H.T.; REX, R.O. and SMITH, J.H.: General observations on the ingrowth of new blood vessels into standardized chambers in the rabbit's ear, and the subsequent changes in newly grown vessels over a period of months. Anat. Rec. *50:* 129–167 (1931).

COMAN, D.R.: Human neoplasms in tissue culture. Cancer Res. *2:* 618–625 (1942).

COOPER, P.: Discussion remarks. Unpublished. Cardiovascular Tissue Culture Conf., Dover, Del., USA (1961).

CURTIS, R.G. and GALVIN, M.P.: Application of a tissue culture technique to screen compounds for the prevention of lipoid deposition in aorta cells. Austr. J. exp. Biol. med. Sci. *41:* 687–694 (1963).

DANIEL, E.E.: Active transport of electrolytes in strips of rabbit aorta and uterus. Arch. int. Pharmacodyn. *158:* 113–130 (1965a). – Effect of sympathomimetic amines and angiotensin on active ion transport in smooth muscle. Arch. int. Pharmacodyn. *158:* 131–138 (1965b).

DANIEL, E.E. and NASH, C.W.: The effects of diuretic and non-diuretic benzothiadiazine and of structurally related diuretic drugs on active ion transport and contractility in smooth muscle. Arch. int. Pharmacodyn. *158:* 139–154 (1965).

DAY, A.J.; NEWMAN, H.A.I. and ZILVERSMIT, D.B.: Synthesis of phospholipid by foam cells isolated from rabbit atherosclerotic lesions. Circulat. Res. *19:* 122–131 (1966).

DETERLING, R.A., JR.; PARSHLEY, M.S. and BLUNT, J.W.: A critical study of present criteria governing selection and use of blood vessel grafts. Surgery *33:* 215–232 (1953).

DUNCAN, L.E., JR. and BUCK, K.: Passage of labeled cholesterol into the aortic wall of the normal dog. Circulat. Res. *7:* 765–770 (1959). – Passage of labeled albumin into canine aortic wall *in vivo* and *in vitro*. Amer. J. Physiol. *200:* 622–624 (1961).

DUNCAN, L.E., JR.; BUCK, K. and LYNCH, A.: Lipoprotein movements through canine aortic wall. Science *142:* 972–973 (1963).

DUNCAN, L.E., JR.; CORNFIELD, J. and BUCK, K.: Circulation of labeled albumin through the aortic wall of the dog. Circulat. Res. *7:* 390–397 (1959). – The effect of blood pressure on the passage of labelled plasma albumin into canine aortic wall. J. clin. Invest. *41:* 1537–1545 (1962).

EAGLE, H.: Nutrition needs of mammalian cells in tissue culture. Science *122:* 501–504 (1955). – Amino acid metabolism in mammalian cell cultures. Science *130:* 432–437 (1959).

EARLE, W.R.; SCHILLING, E.L.; STARK, T.H.; STRAUS, N.P.; BROWN, M.F. and SHELTON, E.: Production of malignancy *in vitro*. IV. The mouse fibroblast cultures and changes seen in living cells. J. nat. Cancer Inst. *4:* 165–212 (1943–44).

EHRENPREIS, S.; BIGO-GULLINO, M. and AVERY, M.A.: The effect of cholinesterase inhibitors and lipid soluble quaternary ammonium compounds on contraction of rabbit aortic strips. Arch. int. Pharmacodyn. *156:* 1–21 (1965).

EISLEY, N.F. and PRITHAM, G.H.: Arterial synthesis of cholesterol *in vitro* from labeled acetate. Science *122:* 121 (1955).

ENGEL, A.F. and POLLAK, O.J.: Free amino acid patterns and other chemical constituents of rabbits' blood and blood vessels. Experientia *17:* 210–211 (1961 b).

ENGEL, A.M.F.: Free amino acid patterns in rabbits' cardiovascular tissue cultures. Unpublished. Cardiovascular Tissue Culture Conf., Dover, Del., USA (1961).

ENGEL, A.M. and POLLAK, O.J.: Free amino acids in media from *in vitro* cultures of normal and atherosclerotic rabbits' aortae. Fed. Proc. *20:* (I) 152 (1961 a).

EVANS, S.M.; IHRIG, H.K.; MEANS, J.A.; ZEIT, W. and HAUSHALTER, E.R.: Atherosclerosis. An *in vitro* study of the pathogenesis of atherosclerosis. Amer. J. clin. Path. *22:* 354–363 (1952).

EVANS, S.M.; MOUNTAIN, D.; BROWN, K.D.; IHRIG, H.K.; ZEIT, W. and HAUSHALTER, E.R.: An *in vitro* study of atherogenesis in rabbits. Abstract. Circulation *12:* 488–489 (1955).

EVANS, V.J.; BRYANT, J.C.; FIORAMONTI, M.C.; MCQILKIN, W.T.; SANFORD, K.K. and EARLE, W.R.: Studies of nutrient media for tissue culture cells *in vitro*. I. A protein-free chemically defined medium for cultivation of strain L-cells. Cancer Res. *16:* 77–86 (1956).

FABRIZIO, A.M.: Biologic membranes as heart valve substitutes. Unpublished. Cardiovascular Tissue Culture Conf., Dover, Del., USA (1961).

FELLER, D.D. and HUFF, R.L.: Lipide synthesis by arterial and liver tissue obtained from cholesterol-fed and cholesterol-alcohol-fed rabbits. Amer. J. Physiol. *182:* 237–242 (1955).

FLORENTIN, R.A.; CHOI, B.H. and NAM, S.C.: DNA synthesis in primary cultures of swine aorta under hypercholesterolemic conditions. Fed. Proc. *27:* 576 (1968).

FLORENTIN, B.H.; CHOI, B.H.; LEE, K.T. and THOMAS, W.A.: Stimulation of DNA synthesis and cell division *in vitro* by serum from cholesterol-fed swine. J. Cell Biol. *41:* 641–645 (1969).

FONTAINE, R.; MANDEL, P.; PONTESCO, V. and KEMPF, E.: The metabolism of the arterial wall and its variations during the ageing process. J. cardiovasc. Surg. *1:* 605–615 (1960).

FOSTER, D.W. and SIPERSTEIN, M.D.: Effects of diabetes on cholesterol and fatty acid synthesis in the rat aorta. Amer. J. Physiol. *198:* 25–28 (1960).

FREEMAN, L. and MORRISON, L. M.: Lipid-clearing effect of acid mucopolysaccharide extract on arterial tissue. Unpublished. Cardiovascular Tissue Culture Conf., Dover, Del., USA (1961).

FRITZ, K. E.; DAOUD, A. S. and JARMOLYCH, J.: Fate of cells in pig aortic medial explants. Fed. Proc. *28:* 681 (1969).

GEER, J. C.: Discussion remarks. Unpublished. Cardiovascular Tissue Culture Conf., Dover, Del., USA (1961).

GEY, G. O. and GEY, M. K.: The maintenance of human normal cells and tumor cells in continuous culture. I. Preliminary report; cultivation of mesoblastic tumors and normal tissue and notes on methods of cultivation. Amer. J. Cancer *27:* 45–76 (1936).

GEYER, R. P.: Uptake and retention of fatty acids by tissue culture cells; in G. H. ROTHBLAT and D. KRITCHEVSKY, Lipid metabolism and tissue culture cells, pp. 33–44 (Wistar Institute Symposium Monograph No. 6, 1967).

GLAGOV, S.; ROWLEY, D. A. and WOLINSKY, H.: Connective tissue layers resembling arterial media formed around implanted pulsating tubes. Abstract. Amer. J. Path. *52:* 25a–26a (1968a). – Pulsating tubes induce tissue growth, J. amer. med. Ass. *205:* 29 (1968b).

GOLDBERG, L. and MORANTZ, D. J.: An *in vitro* study of lipid infiltration of the thick aorta. J. Path. Bact. *74:* 1–15 (1957).

GONZALES, I. E.: Enzyme defects in the diseased arterial wall; in R. J. JONES, Evolution of the atherosclerotic plaque, p. 159 (University of Chicago Press, Chicago, Ill. 1963a). – Cellular metabolic units in atheromatous lesions. Abstract. Circulation *28:* 656 (1963b).

GUTSTEIN, W. J.; LAZZARINI-ROBERTSON, A., JR. and LATAILLADE, J. N.: The role of local arterial irritability in the development of arterio-atherosclerosis. Amer. J. Path. *42:* 61–71 (1963).

HAIMOVICI, H. and MAIER, N.: Role of arterial susceptibility in experimental canine atherosclerosis. J. Atheroscler. Res. *6:* 62–74 (1966).

HANKS, J. H. and WALLACE, R. E.: Relation of oxygen and temperature in the preservation of tissues by refrigeration. Proc. Soc. exp. Biol., N.Y. *71:* 196–200 (1949).

HARARY, I.; GERSCHENSON, L. E.; HAGGERTY, D. F.; DESMOND, W. and MEAD, J. F.: Fatty acid metabolism and function in cultured heart and HeLa cells; in G. H. ROTHBLAT and D. KRITCHEVSKY, Lipid metabolism and tissue culture cells, pp. 17–30 (Wistar Institute Symposium Monograph No. 6, 1967).

HARRISON, R. G.: Observation on the living developing nerve fibre. Proc. Soc. exp. Biol., N.Y. *4:* 140–143 (1907).

HASHIMOTO, S. and DAYTON, S.: Transfer of cholesterol and cholesteryl esters into wall of rat aorta *in vitro*. J. Atheroscler. Res. *6:* 580–590 (1966).

HASTINGS, S. G.; BOOTH, N. H. and HOPWOOD, M. L.: Influence of sex hormones on mucopolysaccharide synthesis of swine arteries. J. Atheroscler. Res. *8:* 29–35 (1968).

HAUST, D.: Discussion remarks. Unpublished. Cardiovascular Tissue Culture Conf., Dover, Del., USA (1961).

HENRY, J. C.: Incorporation d'acides aminés marqués dans des fractions acellulaires de tissu aortique de lapin. Bull. Soc. Chim. biol. *45:* 1413–1421 (1963).

HERZOG, G. und SCHOPPER, W.: Über das Verhalten der Blutgefässe in der Kultur. Arch. exp. Zellforsch. *11:* 202–218 (1931).

HIGGINBOTHAM, A.C.: Observation on normal and atherosclerotic aortic homotransplants in rabbit anterior eye chamber. Anat. Rec. *127:* 308 (1957a). – Intraocular arterial homotransplants for studying atherosclerotic lesion regression. Science *125:* 554–555 (1957b).

HIGGINBOTHAM, A.C. and HIGGINBOTHAM, F.H.: Spontaneous regression in rabbit intraocular atheromatous aortic homotransplants. Arch. Path. *65:* 631–635 (1958).

HRŮZA, Z., BABICKÝ, A. and HLAVÁČKOVÁ, V.: Binding of cholesterol to the rat aorta and collagen fibers during ageing and atherosclerosis *in vitro*. Exp. Geront. *2:* 101–107 (1967).

INGENITO, E.F.; CRAIG, J.M.; LABASSE, J.; GAUTIER, M. and RUTSTEIN, D.D.: Cells of human heart and aorta grown in tissue culture. Arch. Path. *65:* 355–359 (1958).

JENSEN, J.: An *in vitro* method for the study of cholesterol uptake at the endothelial cell surface of the rabbit aorta. Biochim. biophys. Acta *135:* 532–543 (1967a). – The kinetics of the *in vitro* cholesterol uptake at the endothelial cell surface of the rabbit aorta. Biochim. biophys. Acta *135:* 544–556 (1967b).

KAO, V.C.Y.; WISSLER, R.W. and DZOGA, K.: The influence of hyperlipemic serum on the growth of medial smooth muscle cells of rhesus monkey aorta *in vitro*. Abstract. Circulation Suppl. 6 ad *38:* VI–12 (1968).

KASAI, T. and POLLAK, O.J.: Smooth muscle cells in aortic cultures of untreated and cholesterol-fed rabbits. Z. Zellforsch. *62:* 743–752 (1964a). – Action of cigarette smoke on rabbits' cardiovascular cells *in vitro*. Tohoku J. exp. Med. *83:* 245–252 (1964b).

KASAI, T.; POLLAK, O.J. and NAGASAWA, S.: Endothelial cells and macrophages in aortic cultures of untreated and cholesterol-fed rabbits. Z. Zellforsch. *62:* 753–761 (1964).

KIRK, J.E. and LAURSEN, T.J.: Diffusion coefficients of various solutes for human aortic tissue, with special reference to variation in tissue permeability with age. J. Geront. *10:* 288–302 (1955).

KOIDE, R. and POLLAK, O.J.: Phagocytosis by rabbit aortic cells in tissue culture. Unpublished data (1962). – Cytochemical studies of rabbit aortic cells in tissue culture. J. Histochem. Cytochem. *11:* 267–272 (1963a). – The effect of cigarette smoke condensate on rabbits' cardiovascular cells *in vitro*. Exp. molec. Path. *2:* 243–250 (1963b).

KOIDE, R.; POLLAK, O.J. and BURNS, D.: Further observations of aortic cell cultures from untreated and cholesterol-fed rabbits. J. Atheroscler. Res. *3:* 32–43 (1963).

KOKUBU, T.: Aortic and myocardial cells from normo- and hypercholesteremic rabbits. Unpublished. Cardiovascular Tissue Culture Conf., Dover, Del., USA (1961).

KOKUBU, T. and POLLAK, O.J.: Normal rabbits' aortic and myocardial cells grown in various culture media. Abstract. Circulation *22:* 685 (1960). – Normal rabbits' aortic and myocardial cells grown in various culture media. Exp. Cell Res. *24:* 415–423 (1961a). – Tissue cultures of aortae of normal and of cholesterol-fed rabbits. Fed. Proc. *20:* (I) 149 (1961b). – *In vitro* cultures of aortic cells of untreated and of cholesterol-fed rabbits. J. Atheroscler. Res. *1:* 229–239 (1961c). – Influence of nicotine on cells of rabbits' aorta and myocardium in tissue cultures. Exp. molec. Path. *1:* 293–303 (1962).

KOKUBU, T.; POLLAK, O.J. and KOIDE, R.: Comparison of the effect of cigarette-smoke condensate and of nicotine on rabbits' cardiovascular tissue cultures. Abstract. Circulation *24:* 1096 (1961).

KRITSMA, M.G. and BAVINA, M.: Observation on the concentration of essential amino acids demonstrated in some organs and tissues in health and in experimental atherosclerosis (in Russian). Dokl. Akad. Nauk *94:* 721–724 (1954).

LAZZARINI, A.A.: Homoinjertos vasculares conservados. Controlor de valididad por cultivo de tejados. Prensa méd. argent. *39:* 2637–2645 (1952).

LAZZARINI, A.A., JR.: Studies on the absorption of colloidal fat suspensions by vascular cells growing in tissue culture. Abstract. Circulation *12:* 738 (1955). – Studies on the effect of lipoid emulsions on arterial intimal cells in tissue culture in relation to atherosclerosis. Thesis, The Graduate School of Cornell University, 106 pp. (1959).

LAZZARINI, A.A.: Histochemical and electron microscopic studies on cholesterol absorption by human atheromatous plaques. Abstract. Circulation *22:* 656 (1960a).

LAZZARINI, A.A., JR.: Competitive phagocytosis of colloids by arterial intimal cells in tissue culture. Abstract. Excerpta med. *14:* 357 (1960b).

LAZZARINI, A.A., JR. and WEISSMANN, G.: Effects of polyvalent cobalt salts on human cells in tissue culture. Science *131:* 1736–1737 (1960).

LAZZARINI-ROBERTSON, A., JR.: The effects of fatty acids and heparin in the absorption and metabolism of cholesterol microemulsions by organ cultures of human and animal arterial wall; in S. GARATTINI and R. PAOLETTI, Drugs affecting lipid metabolism, pp. 306–313 (Elsevier, Amsterdam 1961a). – Effects of heparin on the uptake of lipids by isolated human and animal endothelial type cells. Angiology, Baltimore *12:* 525–534 (1961b). – Hemodynamic principles and end-to-side anastomosis. Arch. Surg., Chicago *82:* 384–386 (1961c). – Uptake and synthesis of labeled lipoproteins by human and animal arterial organ culture. Unpublished. Cardiovascular Tissue Culture Conf., Dover, Del., USA (1961d). – Effects of oxygen tension on the uptake of labeled lipoproteins by human atheromatous plaques. Abstract. Circulation *24:* 1096–1097 (1961e). – Lipid uptake versus local synthesis in isolated human arterial intima. Abstract. Circulation *26:* 660 (1962a). – The role of local reutilization in atherogenesis. Arch. Surg., Chicago *84:* 41–48 (1962b). – Mechanism of intracellular incorporation of labeled lipids by cloned arterial intimal cells *in vitro.* Abstract. Amer. Soc. Cell Biol., 2nd Ann. Meet., San Francisco, p. 101 (1962c). – Isolation and culture of intimal cells from human and animal arterial wall organ cultures in a chemically defined nutrient. Excerpta med. *16:* 1. Anatomy, 815–816 (1962d). – The role of cholesterol re-utilization in atherogenesis; in B. PRUSÍK, Z. REINIŠ and O. RIEDL, Metabolism parietis vasorum, pp. 42–50 (State Med. Publ. House, Praha 1962e). – Some aspects of the metabolism and ultrastructure of human and animal intimal lining; in S.A. WESOLOWSKI and C. DENNIS, Fundamentals of vascular grafting, pp. 79–105 (McGraw-Hill, London 1963a). – Human pre-atherosclerosis and aging. Abstract. Excerpta med. *57:* 107 (1963b). – Hypoxia and sterol synthesis in human atheromatous plaques. Fed. Proc. *22:* 161 (1963c). – The uptake of labelled lipoproteins by isolated human and animal endothelial type cells; in E.C. HORNING and P. LINDGREN, Effects of drugs on synthesis and mobilization of lipids; Vol. 2, pp. 193–209 (Pergamon Press, Oxford 1963d). – Oxygen requirements of the human arterial intima in atherogenesis. Progr. biochem. Pharmacol., Vol. 4, pp. 305–316 (Karger, Basel/New York 1968).

LEWIS, G.K.: Lipfanogens and antilipfanogens (assayed by tissue cultures) in blood sera of 690 persons, including over 200 patients with 'atherosclerosis'. Unpublished. Cardiovascular Tissue Culture Conf., Dover, Del., USA (1961).

LEWIS, W.H.: The outgrowth of endothelium and capillaries in tissue culture. Johns Hopk. Hosp. Bull. *48:* 242–253 (1931).

LOFLAND, H.B., JR. and CLARKSON, T.B.: Certain metabolic patterns of atheromatous pigeon aortas. Arch. Path. *80:* 291–296 (1965).

LOFLAND, H.B., JR.; CLARKSON, T.B. and ARTOM, C.: Lipide synthesis in aorta preparation from atherosclerosis-susceptible or resistant pigeons. Arch. Biochem. *88:* 105–109 (1960).

LOFLAND, H.B., JR.; MOURY, D.M.; HOFFMAN, C.W. and CLARKSON, T.B.: Lipid metabolism in pigeon aorta during atherogenesis. J. Lipid Res. *6:* 112–118 (1965).

MACKENZIE, D.C. and LOEWENTHAL, J.: Endothelial growth in nylon vascular grafts. Brit. J. Surg. *48:* 212–217 (1960).

MAIER, N. and HAIMOVICI, H.: Oxidative capacity of atherosclerotic tissue of rabbit and dog, with special reference to succinic dehydrogenase and cytochrome oxidase. Circulat. Res. *16:* 65–73 (1965).

MALINOW, M.R.: *In vitro* effect of estradiol on the aorta of chicken. Circulat. Res. *8:* 506–508 (1960).

MAXIMOW, A.: Über die Entwicklungsfähigkeiten der Blutleukozyten und des Blutgefässendothels bei Entzündung und in Gewebskulturen. Klin. Wschr. *4:* 1486–1488 (1925).

MAXWELL, R.A.; WASTILA, W.B. and ECKHARDT, S.B.: Some factors determining the response of rabbit aortic strips to dl-Norepinephrine-7-H^3 hydrochloride and the influence of cocaine, guanethidine and methylphenidate on these factors. J. Pharmacol. exp. Ther. *151:* 253–261 (1966).

MILLER, A.W., JR. and LARSON, P.S.: Observations of the metabolism of nicotine by tissue slices. J. Pharmacol. exp. Ther. *109:* 218–222 (1953).

MORGAN, J.F.; MORTON, H.J. and PARKER, R.C.: Nutrition of animal cells in tissue culture. I. Initial studies on a synthetic medium. Proc. Soc. exp. Biol., N.Y. *73:* 1–8 (1950).

MORRISON, L.M.; MURATA, K.; QUILLIGAN, J.J., JR.; SCHJEIDE, O.A. and FREEMAN, L.: Growth stimulating effects of acid mucopolysaccharides. Proc. Soc. exp. Biol., N.Y. *118:* 770–772 (1965a).

MORRISON, L.M.; SCHJEIDE, O.A.; QUILLIGAN, J.J., JR.; FREEMAN, L. and HOLEMAN, R.: Effects of acid mucopolysaccharides on growth rates and constituent lipids of tissue cultures. Proc. Soc. exp. Biol., N.Y. *113:* 362–366 (1963).

MORRISON, L.M.; SCHJEIDE, O.A.; QUILLIGAN, J.J., JR.; FREEMAN, L. and MURATA, K.: Metabolic parameters of the growth stimulating effect of chondroitin sulfate A in tissue cultures. Proc. Soc. exp. Biol., N.Y. *119:* 618–622 (1965b).

MOSKOWITZ, M.S.: Fatty acid-induced steatosis in monolayer cell cultures; in G.H. ROTHBLAT and D. KRITCHEVSKY, Lipid metabolism and tissue culture cells, pp. 49–59 (Wistar Institute Monograph No. 6, 1967).

MURATA, K.: Synthesis and transport of cholesterol in aortic cells; radioisotopic studies in cell culture. Experientia *24:* 1111–1112 (1968).

MURATA, K.; QUILLIGAN, J.J., JR. and MORRISON, L.M.: Growth of chick aortic endothelial cells: Incorporation of tritiated uridine and thymidine. Experientia *21:* 637–638 (1965). – Relation of aging to metabolism of chick aorta cells: A new approach to the study of aging process and atherosclerosis at the cellular level. Proc. 7th Int. Congr. Gerontology, Vienna, pp. 145–148 (1966). – Suppressing effects of histamine on lipid synthesis in chick aortic cells. Nature, Lond. *213:* 1030–1031 (1967a). – Inhibition of lipid synthesis by puromycin in chick aortic cells. Biochim. biophys. Acta *144:* 473–475 (1967b).

MURRAY, M.R. and STOUT, A.P.: Cultural characteristics of a hemangioendothelioma. Amer. J. Path. *20:* 277–283 (1944).

NAKATANI, M.; SASAKI, T.; MIYAZAKI, T. and NAKAMURA, M.: Synthesis of phospholipids in arterial wall. I. Incorporation of 32-P into phospholipids of aortas and coronary arteries of various animals. J. Atheroscler. Res. *7:* 747–757 (1967a). – Synthesis of phospholipids in arterial wall. II. Effects of age and the addition of adrenalin and acetylcholine on the incorporation of 32-P into phospholipid of rat aorta. J. Atheroscler. Res. *7:* 759–766 (1967b).

NELSON, W.R. and WERTHESSEN, N.T.: Transport of lipids from calf aorta to blood. Abstract. Circulation *18:* 485 (1958).

NEWMAN, H.A.I.; DAY, A.J. and ZILVERSMIT, D.B.: *In vitro* phospholipid synthesis in normal and atheromatous rabbit aortas. Circulat. Res. *19:* 132–138 (1966).

O'NEAL, R.M.; JORDAN, G.L., JR.; RABIN, E., JR.; BAKEY, M.E. DE and HALPERT, B.: Cells grown on isolated intravascular dacron hub. An electron microscopic study. Exp. molec. Path. *3:* 403–412 (1964).

PARKER, R.C.: The races that constitute the group of common fibroblasts. III. Differences determined by origin of explant and age of donor. J. exp. Med. *58:* 401–414 (1933).

PARSHLEY, M.S. and DETERLING, R.A., JR.: The effect of storage at low temperatures on growth *in vitro* of adult dog aorta. Anat. Rec. *115:* 357 (1953). – Tissue culture studies on blood vessel grafts. II. The effect of storage at low temperatures on growth *in vitro* of adult dog aorta. Amer. J. Anat. *97:* 359–394 (1955).

PARSHLEY, M.S.; DETERLING, R.A., JR. and COLEMAN, C.C., JR.: Cultivation *in vitro* of fresh and frozen segments of the abdominal aorta of the dog. Anat. Rec. *106:* 64 (1950). – Tissue culture studies of blood vessel grafts. I. The cultivation *in vitro* of fresh normal adult aorta (dog, cat, rabbit, goat, monkey, and human). Amer. J. Anat. *93:* 221–272 (1953).

PEIRCE, E.C., II.: Preservation of endothelium in refrigerated aortic segments and in aortic homografts in dogs as shown by silver staining. Anat. Rec. *112:* 831–841 (1952).

PEIRCE, E.C., II.; GROSS, R.E.; BILL, A.H., JR. and MERRILL, K., JR.: Tissue culture evaluation of the viability of blood vessels stored by refrigeration. Ann. Surg. *129:* 333–348 (1949).

POLLAK, O.J.: Correlation between chemical and morphologic alterations in experimental atherosclerosis. Arch. Path. *39:* 11–15 (1945). – Visceral atherosclerosis in rabbit and in man. Geriatrics *8:* 135–141 (1953a). – The arteriopathies. II. Atherosclerosis. Unpublished. Lectures to Med. Students (1953b). – Nicotine and cigarette smoke condensate applied to rabbits' cardiovascular cells *in vitro*. Unpublished. Cardiovascular Tissue Culture Conf., Dover, Del., USA (1961). – Elucidation of atherogenesis by cardiovascular cell culture. Mal. cardiovasc. *4:* 29–34 (1963). – Experimental arteriopathies in the rabbit; in J.C. ROBERTS, JR. and R. STRAUSS, Comparative atherosclerosis, pp. 291–310 (Hoeber, New York 1965). – Áterosclerosis en conejo. Colesterol extracirculatorio experimental. Rev. oto-neuro-oftal. Sud-Amer. *42:* 54–57 (1967). – Recent advances in the metabolism of arteries. Tissue cultures, homogenates and slices. Progr. biochem. Pharmacol., Vol. 4, pp. 265–269 (Karger, Basel/New York 1968a). – Cultivo de tejidos en aterosclerosis. Actas IIIer Congr. Interamer. de Ateroscler., Buenos Aires 1968. Rev. oto-neuro-oftal. Sud-Amer. *43:* (Spec. No.) 40–42 (1968b).

POLLAK, O.J. and ADACHI, M.: Human and rabbit arterial cells compared in tissue cultures. Progr. biochem. Pharmacol., Vol. 4, pp. 294–304 (Karger, Basel/New York 1968).

POLLAK, O.J. and BURNS, D.A.: Tissue cultures in cardiovascular research. Motion picture; color and sound; 794 foot, 16 mm, 20 min (1965).

POLLAK, O.J. and KASAI, T.: Identification of spindle cells in tissue cultures of rabbits' aortae. Fed. Proc. *22:* 372 (1963). – Appearance and behavior of aortic cells *in vitro*. Amer. J. med. Sci. *248:* 105–112 (1964).

POLLAK, O.J. and KOKUBU, T.: Effect of nicotine on rabbits' normal and diseased cardiovascular tissue cultures. Fed. Proc. *20:* 149 (1961).

POLLAK, O.J. and WADA, A.: Comparison of *in vivo* and *in vitro* cultures of rabbit aorta. Abstract. Circulation Suppl. 3 ad *34:* 26 (1966). – Extracirculatory cholesterol-atherosclerosis in rabbits. Abstract. Amer. J. Path. *50:* 4a (1967). – *In vivo* aggregation of *in vitro* cultured cells. 7th Int. Congr. Int. Acad. Path., Milano, p. 272 (1968a). – Trauma as a factor in extracirculatory atherosclerosis. Abstract. 7th Int. Congr. Int. Acad. Path., Milano, p. 273 (1968b). – Comparison of *in vivo* and *in vitro* cultures of rabbits' aortae. Abstract. 7th Int. Congr. Int. Acad. Path., Milano, p. 274 (1968c).

POLLAK, O.J.; ENGEL, A.F.; KOKUBU, T. and MORROW, P.: Amino acid patterns in healthy and diseased aortae of rabbits. New approaches to the study of aging and of atherosclerosis. Abstract. 5th Int. Congr. Gerontology, San Francisco, 1960.

POLLAK, O.J.; KOIDE, R. and BURNS, D.A.: Identification of cells in a mixed *in vitro* population from vascular tissue. Fed. Proc. *21:* 2765 (1962a). – Aortic cells *in vitro* as phagocytes. Abstract. Circulation *24:* 667 (1962b).

PRIEST, R.E. and KOPLITZ, R.M.: Inhibition of synthesis of sulfated mucopolysaccharides by estradiol. J. exp. Med. *116:* 565–574 (1962).

PRIEST, R.E. and PRIEST, J.H.: Redifferentiation of connective tissue cells in serial cultures. Science *145:* 1053–1054 (1964).

PRIEST, R.E.; KOPLITZ, R.M. and BENDITT, E.P.: Estradiol reduces incorporation of radioactive sulfate into cartilage and aortae of rats. J. exp. Med. *112:* 225–236 (1960).

PUCK, T.T.; CIECIURA, S.J. and ROBINSON, A.: Genetics of somatic mammalian cells. III. Long-term cultivation of euploid cells from human and animal subjects. J. exp. Med. *108:* 945–955 (1958).

RABINOWITZ, J.L. and RIEMENSCHNEIDER, R.W.: Lipid composition and lipogenesis of intimal areas from a single human aorta. Lab. Invest. *12:* 549–553 (1963).

RIENHOFF, W.F., JR.: Development and growth of the metanephros or permanent kidney in chick embryo (8 to 10 days' incubation). Johns Hopk. Hosp. Bull. *33:* 392–406 (1922).

ROBERTSON, A. L., JR.: Metabolism and ultrastructure of the arterial wall in atherosclerosis. Cleveland Clin. Quart. *32:* 99–117 (1965a). – Intracellular incorporation of plasma lipoproteins by arterial intima in relation to early stages of intravascular thrombosis; in P. SAWYER, Biophysical mechanism in vascular homeostasis and intravascular thrombosis, pp. 267–274 (Appleton-Century-Crofts, New York 1965b). – Selective isolation of cell monolayers from mammalian organ cultures for metabolic studies. Abstract. *In vitro 3:* 174 (Williams and Wilkins, Baltimore 1967a). – Transport of plasma lipoproteins and ultrastructure of human arterial intimacytes in culture; in G.H. ROTHBLAT and D. KRITCHEVSKY, Lipid metabolism and tissue culture cells, pp. 115–125 (Wistar Institute Symposium Monograph 6, 1967b). – Effects of chlorphenoxyisobutyrate on lipid incorporation at cell level. Abstract. Circulation Suppl. 6 ad *38:* VI–20 (1968a). – Differences in lipid metabolism between human xanthoma and atheroma cells. Abstract. Circulation Suppl. 6 ad *38:* VI–20 (1968b); Fed. Proc. *28:* 682 (1969).

ROTHBLAT, G.H. and KRITCHEVSKY, D.: The metabolism of free and esterified cholesterol in tissue culture cells. A review. Exp. molec. Path. *8:* 314–329 (1968).

ROTHBLAT, G.H.; HARTZELL, R.W., JR.; MIALHE, E. and KRITCHEVSKY, D.: The uptake of cholesterol by L 5178Y tissue culture cells; studies with free cholesterol. Biochim. biophys. Acta *116:* 133–145 (1966). – Cholesterol metabolism in tissue culture cells; in G.H. ROTHBLAT and D. KRITCHEVSKY, Lipid metabolism and tissue culture cells, pp. 129–146 (Wistar Institute Monograph No. 6, 1967).

RUTSTEIN, D.D.; CASTELLI, W.P. and NICKERSON, R.J.: Effect of carbohydrate ingestion in humans on intracellular lipid deposition in tissue culture. Amer. J. clin. Nutr. *20:* 98–107 (1967).

RUTSTEIN, D.D.; CASTELLI, W.P.; SULLIVAN, J.C.; NEWELL, J.M. and NICKERSON, R.J.: Effects of fat and carbohydrate ingestion on serum lipids and intracellular lipid deposition in tissue culture. New Engl. J. Med. *271:* 1–11 (1964).

RUTSTEIN, D.D.; INGENITO, E.F.; CRAIG, J.M. and MARTINELLI, M.: Effects of linolenic and stearic acids on cholesterol-induced lipoid deposition in human aortic cells in tissue culture. Lancet 545–552 (1958).

SASAKI, T.; NAKATANI, M. and NAKAMURA, M.: The rate of respiration and incorporation of ^{32}-P into adenosine triphosphate by rat aorta tissue. Jap. Circulat. J. *29:* 1–5 (1965).

SCHWENK, E. and WERTHESSEN, N.T.: Studies on the histogenesis of cholesterol. III. Purification of C^{14}-cholesterol from perfusations of livers and other organs. Arch. Biochem. *40:* 334–341 (1952).

SCRIBA, K.: Explantationsstudien über das Gefäßwachstum bei 9 Tage alten Hühnerembryonen. Arch. exp. Zellforsch. *17:* 68–77 (1935).

SEEGERS, W.: Discussion remarks. Unpublished. Cardiovascular Tissue Culture Conf., Dover, Del., USA (1961).

SHIBUYA, T.: On the pure cultivation of endothelial cells from aorta and their differentiation. Kitasato Arch. exp. Med. *8:* 68–88 (1931).

SILBERBERG, M.: Endothel in der Gewebskultur. Arch. exp. Zellforsch. *9:* 36–53 (1929).

SIMMS, H.S.: The effects of physiologic agents on adult tissues *in vitro*. Science *83:* 418–419 (1936). – A review of research on lipfanogens and antilipfanogen. J. Geront. *6:* 159–162 (1951). – Report on lipfanogen studies in tissue culture. Unpublished. Cardiovascular Tissue Culture Conf., Dover, Del., USA (1961).

SIMMS, H.S. and HARMISON, C.R.: The lipfanogen-antilipfanogen system in relation to lipoproteins, diabetes and species. Angiology, Baltimore, *17:* 872–881 (1966).

SIMMS, H.S. and SANDERS, M.: Use of serum ultrafiltrate in tissue culture for studying deposition of fat and for propagation of viruses. Arch. Path. *33:* 619–635 (1942).

SIMMS, H.S. and STILLMAN, N.P.: Production of fat granules and of degeneration in cultures of adult tissue by agents from blood plasma. Arch. Path. *23:* 316–331 (1937a). – Fat deposition in arteries treated *in vitro* with B factor. Arch. Path. *23:* 332–337 (1937b). – Substances affecting adult tissue *in vitro.* I. The stimulating action of trypsin on fresh adult tissue. J. gen. Physiol. *20:* 603–620 (1937c). – Substances affecting adult tissue *in vitro.* II. A growth inhibitor in adult tissue. J. gen. Physiol. *20:* 621–629 (1937d). – Substances affecting adult tissue *in vitro.* III. A stimulant (the 'A' factor) in serum ultrafiltrate involved in overcoming adult tissue dormancy. J. gen. Physiol. *20:* 649–662 (1937e).

SIMMS, H.S.; HARMISON, C.R. and BEST, R.G.: Cholesterol and antilipfanogen in arteriosclerosis. J. Geront. *9:* 133–141 (1954).

SIMMS, H.S.; LINDGREN, F.T.; HARMISON, C.R.; NICHOLS, A.V. and MURAVIEW, T.: Lipfanogen and antilipfanogen determinations on serum lipoprotein fractions. Lab. Invest. *5:* 162–174 (1956).

SIMMS, H.S.; PARSHLEY, M.S. and PITT, R.B.: Fat deposition *in vitro* caused by lipfanogens and opposed by antilipfanogens. J. Geront. *2:* 205–216 (1947).

SIPERSTEIN, M.D.; CHAIKOFF, I.L. and CHERNICK, S.S.: Significance of endogenous cholesterol in arteriosclerosis. Synthesis in arterial tissue. Science *113:* 747–749 (1951).

SMITH, S.C.; STROUT, R.G.; DUNLOP, W.R. and SMITH, E.C.: Fatty acid composition of cultured aortic cells from White Carneau and Show Racer pigeons. J. Atheroscler. Res. *5:* 379–387 (1965).

ST. CLAIR, R.W.; LOFLAND, H.B. and CLARKSON, T.D.: Composition and synthesis of fatty acids in atherosclerotic aortas of the pigeon. J. Lipid Res. *9:* 739–747 (1968a).

ST. CLAIR, R.W.; LOFLAND, H.B., JR.; PRICHARD, R.W. and CLARKSON, T.B.: Synthesis of squalene and sterols by isolated segments of human and pigeon arteries. Exp. molec. Path. *8:* 201–215 (1968b).

STEIN, Y. and STEIN, O.: Incorporation of fatty acids into lipids of aortic slices of rabbits, dogs, rats and baboons. J. Atheroscler. Res. *2:* 400–412 (1962).

STEIN, Y.; STEIN, O. and SHAPIRO, B.: Enzymic pathways of glyceride and phospholipid synthesis in aortic homogenates. Biochim. biophys. Acta *70:* 33–42 (1963).

STRONG, J.P.; MCGILL, H.C., JR. and NYMAN, M.A.: Deposition of lipid in calf aorta maintained *in vitro.* Circulat. Res. *5:* 294–297 (1957).

STUMP, M.M.; JORDAN, G.L., JR.; BAKEY, M.E. DE and HALPERT, B.: The endothelial lining of homografts and dacron prosthesis in the canine aorta. Amer. J. Path. *40:* 487–491 (1962). – Endothelium grown from circulating blood on isolated dacron hub. Amer. J. Path. *43:* 361–367 (1963).

SWAN, H.; FEEHAN, J.J.; FLORIO, L. and JOHNSON, R.T.: Arterial homografts. IV. Preservation of tissue culture viability of canine aortic segments after freezing at low temperatures. Surgery *31:* 807–820 (1952).

TÖRÖ, E.: Untersuchungen über die Potenz der Endothelzellen bei der Gefäßbildung in der Gewebskultur. Arch. exp. Zellforsch. *20:* 156–171 (1937).

TUME, R.K., BRADLEY, T.R. and DAY, A.J.: An investigation by tissue culture techniques on the growth of foam cells isolated from rabbit. J. Atheroscler. Res. *9:* 151–157 (1969).

WADA, A. and POLLAK, O.J.: Aggregation *in vivo* of cultured aortic cells of adult rabbits. Nature, Lond. *214:* 1358–1360 (1967a). – Extracirculatory atherosclerosis in rabbits. Arch. Path. *84:* 460–467 (1967b). – *In vivo* organ reconstruction from cells cultured *in vitro*. Cell Tissue Kin. *2:* 39–46 (1969).

WAYMOUTH, C.: Rapid proliferation of NCTC clone 929 (strain L) mouse cells in a simple chemically defined medium (MB 752/1). J. nat. Cancer Inst. *22:* 1003–1017 (1959). – Construction and use of synthetic media; in E.N. WILLMER, Cells and tissues in culture. Methods, biology and physiology, Vol. 1, pp. 118–119 (Academic Press, London/New York 1965).

WERTHESSEN, N.T.: Chemical agents capable of affecting lipid metabolism in the aorta. Circulat. Res. *6:* 759–764 (1958). – Control of aortal lipid metabolism and lipid movement by hormones and vitamins; in G. PINCUS, Hormones and atherosclerosis, pp. 131–141 (Academic Press, New York 1959). – Studies on aortae maintained *in vitro*. Unpublished, Cardiovascular Tissue Culture Conf., Dover, Del., USA (1961).

WERTHESSEN, N.T.; HAHN, J.W. and NYMAN, M.A.: Lipid and cholesterol synthesis in the perfused calf aorta; in A.C. FRAZER, Biochemical problems of lipids, pp. 401–408 (Elsevier, Amsterdam 1956).

WERTHESSEN, N.T.; MILCH, L.S.; REDMOND, R.F.; SMITH, L.L. and SMITH, E.C.: Biosynthesis and concentration of cholesterol by the intact surviving bovine aorta *in vitro*. Amer. J. Physiol. *178:* 23–29 (1954).

WERTHESSEN, N.T.; NYMAN, N.A.; HOLMAN, R.L. and STRONG, J.P.: *In vitro* study of cholesterol metabolism of the calf aorta. Circulat. Res. *4:* 586–593 (1956).

WERTHESSEN, N.T.; NYMAN, M.; STRONG, J.P. and HOLMAN, R.L.: Factors influencing the biosynthesis of lipids by calf aorta *in vitro*. Abstract. Circulation *12:* 488 (1955).

WEXLER, B. and THOMAS, L.: Growth of aortic explants and arteriosclerosis. Nature, Lond. *214:* 243–245 (1967).

WHITE, J.F. and PARSHLEY, M.S.: Growth *in vitro* of blood vessels from the bone marrow of adult chicken. Amer. J. Anat. *89:* 321–345 (1951).

WILENS, S.L.: The experimental production of lipid deposition in excised arteries. Science *114:* 389–393 (1951).

WILENS, S.L. and MCCLUSKEY, R.T.: The comparative filtration properties of excised arteries and veins. Amer. J. med. Sci. *224:* 540–547 (1952). – The permeability of excised arteries and other tissues to serum lipid. Circulat. Res. *2:* 175–182 (1964).

ZILVERSMIT, D.B.; MCCANDLESS, E.L.; JORDAN, P.H., JR. and ACKERMAN, R.F.: The synthesis of phospholipids in human atheromatous lesions. Circulation *23:* 370–375 (1961).

SUBJECT INDEX

MONOGRAPHS ON ATHEROSCLEROSIS

Volumes in preparation

ENGELBERG. H. (Beverly Hills, CA): Heparin.

HOWARD, A.N. and GRESHAM, G.A. (Cambridge): Primates.

KIRK, J.E. (St. Louis, MO): Enzyme Cofactors in Arterial Tissue.

MUSTARD, J.F.; MURPHY, E.A. and SCHWARTZ, S.J. (Hamilton, Ont.): Blood Platelets.

ROBINSON, R.W. (Worcester, MA): Mucopolysaccharides.

RODBARD, S. (Duarte, CA): Blood Stream and Vascular Structure.

SIMMS, H.S. (Rockleigh, NJ): The Lipfanogen-antilipfanogen System.